Navigating VA Health Care

A Veteran's Guide to Enforcing Your Rights, Fixing the Record, and Holding the VA System Accountable

John Lafferty

Copyright © 2025 by John Lafferty
All rights reserved.

No part of this publication may be reproduced, stored in a retrieval system, or transmitted in any form or by any means—electronic, mechanical, photocopying, recording, or otherwise—without the prior written permission of the author, except for brief quotations used in reviews or permitted by law for educational purposes.

This is an independent work and is not affiliated with, endorsed by, or associated with the U.S. Department of Veterans Affairs (VA), the Veterans Health Administration (VHA), or any government agency.

References to laws, regulations, directives, and handbooks are for educational and advocacy purposes. All cited materials are in the public domain.

Cover design created using AI tools from OpenAI (ChatGPT), with final concept and direction by the author.

Printed in the United States of America

ISBN: 979-8-9997129-0-5

First Edition

Legal Notice

This book is intended for educational and informational purposes only and does not constitute legal, medical, or professional advice. The author is not affiliated with the Department of Veterans Affairs (VA), and this guide is not endorsed by any government agency. Readers are encouraged to consult appropriate legal or medical professionals when addressing personal health care or benefits decisions.

References to VA policies, directives, or federal law are accurate to the best of the author's knowledge at the time of publication but are subject to change. Always verify current VA regulations before taking formal action.

About This Book

Navigating the VA health care system can be overwhelming, confusing, and exhausting — even for those who served with honor. This guide was created as a practical, plain-language tool for Veterans, caregivers, advocates, and VA staff who want to understand how the system is designed to work — and how to hold it accountable when it falls short.

There are countless resources on winning VA disability claims, but few explain what comes after the rating decision — the daily reality of accessing care, overcoming barriers, and asserting your rights within the VA health system. This guide is based on real-world experience, deep research into VA policies, federal law, and years of personal advocacy. Every rule, directive, and regulation cited here comes directly from the VA's own playbook.

This book doesn't encourage conflict; it equips you to advocate effectively. By understanding your rights and the VA's legal obligations, you gain the tools to act when the system fails to meet its own standards. The goal is simple: to empower Veterans with the tools they need to get the care they earned — and deserve.

▌ How to Use This Book

This book is a toolset for Veterans, caregivers, and advocates who need more than encouragement — they need results. Whether you're new to VA health care or have spent years fighting the system, this guide gives you the information, leverage, and language to respond effectively — and in writing.

You don't need to read this book in order. Use the Table of Contents to jump directly to what you need. Every chapter is built to stand alone, with cross-references to supporting material and appendices.

Here's how to get the most from it:

🔑 If You're Facing Delays, Denials, or Disrespect

Jump to:

- **Chapter 8** – *When Patient Advocates Don't Do Their Job*
- **Chapter 10** – *Writing Complaints That Get Results*
- **Appendix C** – *Complaint Templates and Examples*
- **Appendix D** – *Complaint Strategy Quick Reference Table*

These sections are designed for immediate action — even if the VA is ignoring you, these tools help you document the problem and escalate it strategically.

📄 If You Need Records Fixed or Forms Completed

Go to:

- **Chapter 12** – *Your Right to Medical Statements and Form Completion*
- **Chapter 13** – *Amending VA Medical Records*

These sections walk you through how to request completed paperwork, respond to refusals, and legally challenge false or misleading entries in your VA records.

🛠 If You're Ready to Take Action or Escalate

Start with:

- **Part II: Advocacy in Action**
- **Part III: Escalation and Enforcement**
- **Chapter 17** – *Writing to Congress and the VA Secretary*
- **Appendix E** – *Logging VA Contacts and Building Your Paper Trail*

These sections show how to escalate unresolved problems, build a compelling record, and hold staff accountable using the VA's own policies and laws.

👥 If You're Helping Another Veteran

Focus on:

- **Chapter 15** – *Social Work and Advocacy*
- **Chapter 18** – *From Patient to Advocate*

Whether you're a caregiver, friend, or fellow Veteran, these chapters help you become a stronger advocate for someone else — with tips on boundaries, documentation, and backup plans.

📚 If You Want to Understand How the VA Health System Is Supposed to Work

Begin with:

- **Part I – Understanding the System**

Learn what the Patient Advocate Program is legally required to do, how VA health care is structured, and what rights every Veteran is supposed to have — whether the VA follows them or not.

📄 Use the Appendices for Quick Access

These are your strategic toolkit for citing policy, building your case, and documenting VA failures:

- **Appendix A** – *Key VA Directives, Laws, and Regulations Referenced*
- **Appendix B** – *VA Terms Every Veteran Should Know*
- **Appendix C** – *Complaint Templates and Examples*
- **Appendix D** – *Complaint Strategy Quick Reference Table*
- **Appendix E** – *Logging VA Contacts and Building Your Paper Trail*
- **Appendix F** – *Commonly Cited USC, CFR, VHA Directives and Handbooks*

🔑 Final Tip:

When you're not getting help, use this book to create a paper trail. When you're not being heard, use it to escalate. When you're being mistreated, use it to push back. You don't need permission — you need a plan. This book is that plan.

Table of Contents

PART I Understanding the System 1
Chapter 1: Learning the System After the Rating Decision 2
Chapter 2: Understanding How VA Health Care Is Organized.............. 5
Chapter 3: Following the Rules for Veteran Patient Experience 10
Chapter 4: Using Patient Advocates When the System Fails 15

PART II Advocacy in Action..19
Chapter 5: Using VA Policy to Strengthen Your Case 20
Chapter 6: Applying Veteran Experience Policy to Your Situation.........30
Chapter 7: Understanding the Law Behind Patient Advocacy 35
Chapter 8: Responding When Patient Advocates Don't Help 40

PART III Escalation and Enforcement 54
Chapter 9: Escalating Complaints Beyond the Local VA 55
Chapter 10: Writing Complaints That Get Attention..........................64
Chapter 11: Following Up and Maintaining Pressure 78

PART IV Taking Control of the Record 93
Chapter 12: Requesting Medical Statements and Form Completion 94
Chapter 13: Amending False or Misleading VA Medical Records.........107
Chapter 14: Recognizing Hidden Hazards in Your VA Record.............126

PART V Support Systems and Coordinated Care 136
Chapter 15: Using Social Work for Advocacy and Support................137
Chapter 16: Exploring Whole Health and Veteran Empowerment 145
Chapter 17: Navigating Care with Your PACT Team 155

PART VI —Final Thoughts and References............................... 168
Chapter 18: Becoming a Veteran Advocate for Others 169
Chapter 19: Working Toward System-Level Change 172
Chapter 20: Finding Strength in Shared Veteran Experience 175

Appendices 178
Appendix A: Key VA Directives, Laws, and Regulations Referenced ...178
Appendix B: VA Terms Every Veteran Should Know 191

Appendix C: Complaint Templates and Examples 194

Appendix D: Complaint Strategy Quick Reference Table 209

Appendix E: Logging VA Contacts and Building Your Paper Trail 210

Appendix F: Commonly Cited USC, CFR, VHA Directives and Handbooks 212

Appendix G: How to File a Record Amendment 230

Index   237

VA Structure & Entities 237

Legal & Policy References... 238

Complaint & Appeal Mechanisms.. 239

Medical Records... 239

Access & Treatment Issues... 240

Veteran Experience 240

Forms & Communication 241

Accountability & Oversight 241

PART I

Understanding the System

> *"You cannot fight a system you don't understand — and you certainly can't fix one."*

Before you can advocate for better care, write a strong complaint, or hold VA staff accountable, you need to know the system you're working within. That's what this section is about.

Part I lays the foundation. It explains how VA health care is structured, what rules are supposed to guide your experience as a patient, and who's responsible when things go wrong. These chapters are designed to take the mystery out of VA processes and put that knowledge in your hands — not as trivia, but as tools.

You'll learn:

- How the VA health care system is organized and where your facility fits in
- What legal standards define the *Veteran Patient Experience*
- Who Patient Advocates are, what they are supposed to do, and why they matter more than most Veterans realize

If you've ever left a VA appointment feeling dismissed, delayed, or disrespected, you're not alone. But you're also not powerless. The VA doesn't just run on culture — it runs on policy. And once you know those policies, you stop asking for help and start demanding accountability.

This section will give you that starting point — because you can't change what you don't understand.

Chapter 1: Learning the System After the Rating Decision

In some parts of the VA system, tribal knowledge can quietly replace written policy. What gets done — or doesn't — is often shaped more by routine than regulation. These habits can become so deeply ingrained that even supervisors may treat them as truth — not because they're correct, but because they were trained the same way. But repetition doesn't equal legitimacy. That's why knowing the rules — and how to use them — matters more than ever.

Section 1 — Why this book matters

Search the internet and you'll find countless articles, videos, and blogs about how to win VA disability claims and where to go for claims help. Let's face it — winning claims will always be a hot topic, because the system is complicated, confusing, and Veterans know they're losing out on benefits they've earned.

But once those ratings are awarded, what comes next? That's where it gets quiet. This book fills that gap by focusing on what happens after your claim is approved — the real-life challenges inside the VA health system. Not every Veteran struggles with the Veterans Health Administration — or VHA, for short. That wasn't mine. And if you're reading this, I'm guessing it wasn't yours either.

VHA is a huge system with too many moving parts. No one person knows it all — not the doctors, not the social workers, not the Patient Advocates, and not even the folks answering the 800 number. Yes, the VHA Directives, Handbooks, and the 38 U.S.C. laws are all online. But they're written in language that makes sense to the people who wrote them — not to the veterans trying to understand and navigate their own care.

That's why I wrote this guide. Like many Veterans, I've had to fight my way through the VHA — not just to get care, but to get VA employees to follow their own rules. Along the way, I dug deep into the laws, court rulings, directives, and policies that are supposed to govern this system. What you'll find here isn't just advice — it's backed by the same rules VA is required to follow, even if some employees would rather you didn't know them. What you'll find here is backed by VA law, federal regulation, and formal policy — not hearsay or opinion.

If sharing what I've learned helps even one Veteran avoid some of the battles I've faced, this guide will have done its job. And if I can make your path through the Veterans Health Administration even a little bit easier, then writing this book was worth it.

Section 2 — The VA system: strengths and frustrations

With all the complaints about VA health care, some Veterans ask a fair question: *"Why bother with the VA at all?"*

It's a fair question, especially for those who do have the option to choose.

The truth is, VA health care (VHA) has both strengths and frustrations. Not every clinic or hospital runs the same way, and not every Veteran faces the same problems. I've seen VHA facilities that struggle badly, and others that serve Veterans very well. For example, some facilities offer streamlined referrals, quick specialty appointments, and care teams that truly listen. And while there are certainly challenges, I can also tell you this: the VHA has some excellent doctors. At the time of writing this guide, I'm fortunate to have both a strong primary care physician and excellent specialty care providers — though that wasn't always the case.

One key difference between VA health care and the private system is this: VHA staff are legally required to follow a specific set of laws, regulations, and directives — all of which are publicly available. The frustration comes when they don't. But here's where knowledge becomes power. If you know which rules apply and how to cite and apply them — especially in writing— you can compel the system to act correctly. That gives you a level of control most private health care systems simply don't provide.

In this guide, I'll show you how to do exactly that.

Section 3 — Who this guide is for

Veterans and caregivers are already stretched thin. Most lack the time or energy to decode how the VA health care system actually functions — even when they're forced to rely on it. This guide is for any Veteran, spouse, caregiver, or family member who finds themselves stuck, frustrated, or just plain confused about how to get care, who to talk to, or how to get someone to finally listen. Whether you're new to the VA or have been fighting it for years, this guide offers practical advice you can actually use — all backed by the very rules VA staff are supposed to follow. Veteran Service Officers, VA staff, and others working in the system can also benefit. This guide translates dense policy into practical tactics that can help them support Veterans more effectively. Sometimes even well-meaning staff aren't fully aware of the policies, directives, or appeal processes available to Veterans. My hope is that this guide not only helps Veterans advocate for themselves, but also helps those who serve Veterans become stronger advocates as well.

So, let's start at the beginning — because the better you understand how the VA health care system is structured, the more effectively you can make it work for you.

Chapter 2: Understanding How VA Health Care Is Organized

Most Veterans see the VA health care system as a single entity, but in reality, it operates more like a collection of loosely connected parts. Departments often fail to communicate, and when they don't, mistakes follow.

You don't need to be an expert. But you do need to understand how the system is supposed to function. The more you know, the more effectively you can advocate when things go wrong.

Section 1 — The Big Picture: How VA Is Organized

The Department of Veterans Affairs has three primary branches:

- Veterans Benefits Administration (VBA): Handles disability ratings, compensation, pensions.
- Veterans Health Administration (VHA): Provides medical care.
- National Cemetery Administration (NCA): Manages burial and memorial benefits.

Though all fall under the VA umbrella, they often function like separate organizations with limited communication between them — and yes, you're probably thinking that's messed up. You're not wrong. But knowing that upfront won't change how they operate — it'll just help you stay sane.

When engaging with the VA, the most likely order you will encounter them:

- Start with VBA to establish eligibility and ratings.
- Then transition to VHA for your health care.
- Eventually, NCA becomes relevant for burial and memorial services.

Don't assume information shared with one branch is available to another. Always be prepared to submit the same documents multiple times.

Section 2 — Eligibility & Priority Groups: What They Really Mean

When you first step into the VA system, one of the first things they do is figure out if you're eligible for care — and where you fit in the VA's system of access and priority. That's where things like Eligibility and Priority Groups come in.

Eligibility depends on four main factors:

- Length of service
- Discharge status
- Service-connected disability status
- Special circumstances (e.g., combat service, toxic exposures)

If you served honorably and meet the minimum active-duty requirements (usually 24 continuous months if you joined after 1980), you're generally eligible to enroll in VA health care. But that's just step one — next comes your Priority Group, and that's where it gets a little more complicated.

The VA uses Priority Groups (PGs) to sort Veterans into different levels, which affects your access to care and copays. Think of it like being assigned a boarding group at the airport — everyone gets on the plane, but some board sooner than others.

Here's a very basic breakdown:

- **PG 1**: 50%-100% SC, IU, SMC, or Medal of Honor recipients
- **PG 2**: 30%-40% SC
- **PG 3**: 10%-20% SC, Purple Heart, POWs, certain discharges
- **PG 4**: Aid & Attendance, Housebound, catastrophically disabled
- **PG 5**: Low-income, VA pension recipients, Medicaid eligible
- **PG 6**: PACT Act eligible (e.g., toxic exposures)
- **PG 7**: Higher-income but below geographic thresholds
- **PG 8**: No SC and above income thresholds (lowest priority)

Note: Your Priority Group may change if your rating changes. Don't assume this happens automatically — follow up yourself.

The bottom line: the lower your number, the better your access and the fewer copays you'll face. But even lower-level Priority Group Veterans are still eligible for care — you just may have more paperwork, copays, or delays depending on demand at your facility.

Section 3 — The Enrollment Process: How to Get Into VA Health Care

While most readers are probably already enrolled, this section is still worth covering. Some Veterans picking up this guide might be just getting started, or you may find yourself helping as a caregiver, friend, or fellow vet who hasn't made it this far yet.

There are four ways to apply:

1. **Online:** Fastest. Visit choose.va.gov/health.
2. **Phone:** Call 877-222-8387.
3. **In-person:** Visit a VA facility with documentation.
4. **Mail:** Least reliable; risk of document loss.

You will typically need:

- Social Security number
- DD-214
- Private insurance info (if applicable)
- Financial info for means-testing (if needed)

Section 4 — The Parts of VA That Control Your Health Care

The three main pieces where you get care:

- **VA Medical Centers (VAMCs):** Full-service hospitals with specialty clinics, surgeries, and emergency care.
- **Community-Based Outpatient Clinics (CBOCs):** Local clinics for routine care and labs.
- **Community Care:** Private care paid for by VA when VA can't meet your needs.

Think of it this way: CBOCs handle the everyday. VAMCs handle the complex. Community Care fills the gaps.

Section 5 — Primary Care vs. Specialty Care: Who Controls Access to What

In the VA system, your Primary Care Provider (PCP) controls nearly all access to care. They're the gatekeeper. You need a referral for nearly every specialist.

Here's the process:

- PCP submits a consult
- Specialist reviews and accepts/rejects
- Appointment scheduled (if approved)

Breakdowns often happen here. Referrals may be:

- Improperly worded
- Denied silently
- Not followed up on

That's why knowing *how* the system routes referrals gives you leverage. If your PCP doesn't submit the request properly, you won't get seen. If the specialist denies it, you have every right to ask for the reason — and to push back.

We'll cover how to push back on referral delays later in this book. Just know for now: Primary Care is your launchpad. Specialists are your destination. But you control how much you push for takeoff.

Section 6 — Meet Your PACT (Patient Aligned Care Team)

VA loves acronyms, and PACT is one you'll hear a lot. Your Patient Aligned Care Team (PACT) is supposed to be your support crew for everything related to your health care. Your PACT isn't just one doctor — it's an entire care team.

A typical PACT includes:

- **Primary Care Provider (PCP)**: Your main doctor or nurse practitioner.

- **Registered Nurse Care Manager (RNCM)**: Helps coordinate your care, manage chronic conditions, and keep track of follow-ups.

- **Licensed Practical Nurse (LPN)**: Assists with procedures, vitals, and clinic operations.

- **Clerical Associate (Clerk)**: Schedules appointments, handles paperwork, and manages communication between you and the team.

- **Pharmacist / Clinical Social Worker** (depending on need): Help manage medications, home care needs, or social services.

In practice, some PACT teams excel while others barely function. Learn your team members' names. Follow up if things fall through.

The system is designed for coordinated care, but execution varies. Understanding your rights and the VA's obligations is the key to getting the care you earned.

Chapter 3: Following the Rules for Veteran Patient Experience

"*Veteran Patient Experience*" may sound like a buzzword, but don't let the polite phrasing fool you. What it really means is how VA staff are expected to treat you — not just in attitude, but in action. These are the operational standards that VA employees are supposed to follow, written into federal regulations and VA policy. When those standards are ignored, delayed, or twisted into excuses, you're not just dealing with bad service — you're facing a violation of policy. This chapter explains what those rules are, where they come from, and how you can use them to fight back when the system breaks down.

Section 1 — The Rules of the Road: The Laws and Regulations the VA Follows

Let's start with a core truth: VA staff are not free to make up the rules as they go. The VA health care system is governed by a clear legal framework that spells out exactly what should happen at every level — from the front desk clerk to the Medical Center Director.

That framework includes:

- **United States Code (USC):** These are the actual federal laws written by Congress. The 38 U.S.C. covers veteran benefits and health care.

- **Code of Federal Regulations (CFR):** These are the rules federal agencies like the VA write to implement laws. The 38 U.S.C. of the CFR breaks down how VA must apply the laws.

- **VHA Directives:** These are mandatory internal policies that VHA staff must follow. They cover everything from patient rights to referrals to complaint handling.

- **VHA Handbooks and VA Handbooks**: These explain how to carry out the Directives in practice.

Here's why that matters: When something goes wrong with your care, you're not just left with frustration. You have recourse. You have rules on your side — written by the VA itself.

Let me give you a personal example: When my local Patient Advocate office tried to brush off my complaint, they handed me their own "local SOP" (standard operating procedure). But when I presented the actual federal law — 38 U.S.C. § 7309A — and VA policy — VHA Directive 1003.04 — they were caught completely off guard. They had no idea those rules even existed. That moment taught me something critical: sometimes you'll know VA policy better than the people paid to enforce it. And that knowledge changes everything.

Section 2 — The VA's Legal Obligation to Provide Respectful, Effective Service

Let's zoom out. VA policy is important, but it's built on an even stronger foundation: federal law.

According to **38 CFR § 603**, every federal agency — including the VA — must meet certain customer experience principles. This regulation isn't VA marketing fluff. It's binding federal law.

What does that mean for you as a Veteran? You have the legal right to:

- Receive timely, accurate information
- Get decisions explained clearly and in plain language
- Be treated with professionalism and respect
- Expect the VA to use your feedback to improve its service

These aren't nice suggestions. These are binding legal standards federal agencies must follow — right now, not someday.

So, when you face month-long delays, vague explanations, or rude encounters, it's not just bad manners — it's a breakdown in the agency's legal duty. These are not favors you have to beg for. They are standards the VA is required to meet.

Section 3 — VHA Directive 1003: The Core of Veteran Patient Experience Policy

If 38 CFR § 603 sets the legal floor, **VHA Directive 1003** builds the operational structure. This is the VA's own internal policy on what the Veteran Patient Experience is supposed to look like in practice.

VA leadership loves to use phrases like "veteran-centered care," "personalized service," and "Whole Health." While those phrases might trigger involuntary eye-rolls for Veterans with highly tuned BS meters, here's what most don't realize: these words aren't just part of VA's marketing speeches — VHA Directive 1003 turns them into mandatory policy.

VHA Directive 1003 defines how the VA is supposed to fulfill the legal standards laid out in CFR §603. It states that your care must be:

- **Patient-driven:** Your needs and goals come first
- **Proactive:** Problems are supposed to be prevented, not just reacted to
- **Personalized:** Your circumstances should shape your care
- **Coordinated:** All parts of your care team should work together

These are not inspirational posters. This is mandatory policy. Every VA facility is required to:

- Have written procedures to implement these standards
- Assign leadership roles to oversee them
- Train staff regularly
- Use feedback to fix broken systems

In other words, if your care feels disjointed, impersonal, or chaotic, it's not just bad luck. It may be a violation of VHA Directive 1003.

And it doesn't stop there. VHA Directive 1003 also requires:

- **Service Recovery:** When something breaks down, VA staff must take immediate steps to fix it and restore trust.
- **Process Improvement:** VA leaders must track recurring problems and fix system-wide issues to prevent harm.

If you keep hearing "We'll get back to you" or "That's not our department," that's not just poor service. It's a violation of the VA's own policy on Service Recovery.

From now on, when your clinic keeps losing referrals, or your specialty care team constantly delays appointments, or the same communication failures keep happening over and over — VA leadership is already under written policy to track, analyze, and fix these system-wide problems.

VA doesn't get to normalize broken systems. Their own policies require them to prevent repeated failures — not just fix them after you complain.

So, when you hear VA staff say:

- *"That's just how it works here."*
- *"We've always done it this way."*
- *"There's nothing I can do about it."*

You'll know better.

Section 4 — Accountability Isn't Optional: Leadership Has Duties Too

When most Veterans run into problems at the VA, the frustration often starts with whoever is right in front of them — the scheduler who never calls back, the nurse who loses your consult, the specialist who rejects a referral without explanation. While it may seem like the problem stops with the clerk or the scheduler or the nurse, in truth, the real responsibility lies higher up. According to VHA Directives 1003 and 1003.04, Medical Center Directors are personally responsible for ensuring their facility meets these standards. That includes:

- Overseeing the Patient Advocacy Program
- Monitoring complaint data
- Fixing recurring issues

The buck doesn't stop at the front desk. It stops at the Director's desk. And above them? The VISN Director oversees multiple facilities and is responsible for ensuring those Directors do their jobs.

So, when you escalate your concern beyond a clinic, you are not breaking protocol. You are following the accountability chain the VA created.

And here's why it matters even more: VA leadership performance is tied to these standards. Directors are evaluated on things like:

- Patient satisfaction scores
- Complaint resolution
- Service recovery rates

When you escalate unresolved issues, you're doing more than seeking help. You're activating the very system that holds leadership accountable. In other words, you're not being a problem when you escalate — you're using the accountability system VA was legally required to create.

Section 5 — Your VA Health Care Rights: What You're Entitled to Demand

By now, you've seen that VA health care isn't just built on vague promises or nice-sounding mission statements. It's built on law. On written directives. On hard policies that govern every interaction you have with the system. These are not hopes or goals. They are enforceable rules VA staff are obligated to follow — whether they personally know them or not.

- Let's make this personal. As a Veteran receiving VA care, you have the right to:
- Be treated with dignity at every point of contact
- Receive timely referrals, appointments, and responses
- Be given honest, plain-language explanations
- Expect your care team to coordinate behind the scenes
- Receive service recovery when something breaks down
- See broken systems get fixed, not repeated
- Access the Patient Advocate when things go wrong
- Escalate your concerns to leadership when others fail you

And let's be clear: **exercising these rights is not being difficult.** It's demanding the system follow its own rules. The burden of compliance sits with the VA — not you. Their job is to follow their own rulebook. Your job is to know that rulebook exists and how to use it when necessary.

You don't have to be a lawyer to enforce these rights. You just need to know where they live — and how to use them. You've earned these rights through your service. Now it's time to make the VA honor them.

In Chapter 4, we'll dig into the Patient Advocacy Program — what it was created to do, what the law says about its role, and how to respond when it falls short.

Chapter 4: Using Patient Advocates When the System Fails

Veterans don't ask for special treatment. We just expect the system to work the way it says it will. But too often, it doesn't — and when it doesn't, one of the first places you're told to go is the Patient Advocate.

This chapter is not about their legal requirements — we'll cover that in Chapter 7. Instead, this chapter is your field guide to using Patient Advocates strategically. What works, what doesn't, how to approach them, and what to do when they refuse to help.

Section 1 — What Patient Advocates *Should* Be Doing

If the VA system worked smoothly, you'd never need a Patient Advocate. But it doesn't — and that's exactly why this role exists. Patient Advocates are supposed to help when communication breaks down, when appointments fall through, when referrals vanish, and when staff don't listen.

But let's be real: at some facilities, the Patient Advocate just takes notes, forwards the complaint to the service line to be looked at, and hopes for the best. That's not acceptable — and it's not what their job is supposed to be.

In theory, a good Patient Advocate should:

- Listen carefully to your concern
- Take ownership of the problem
- Coordinate with the right department or service line
- Follow up until the issue is resolved
- Notify you of the outcome

Some do. Many don't.

This chapter helps you deal with the ones who don't.

Section 2 — The 3 Rules for Using Patient Advocates Effectively

Here's what I've learned through hard experience:

Rule 1: Document Everything Before You Go In

Don't walk in angry and empty-handed. Walk in prepared. Bring:

- Dates, names, and specific events
- Copies of messages or call logs
- Reference to the directive or policy being violated (you'll learn those throughout this book)

A Patient Advocate is more likely to help if they see you've done your homework and can't be brushed off.

Rule 2: Make a Specific Ask

Don't just say "I'm frustrated." Say:

- *"I need a response from the neurology clinic within 48 hours."*
- *"I want to know why my referral was rejected."*
- *"I need this added to my record: [insert statement]."*

Specific requests get action. Vague complaints get shelved.

Rule 3: If They Won't Act, Escalate

If the Advocate shrugs or says, *"I just log complaints,"* it's time to move up the chain. Don't argue. Ask politely:

- *"Who supervises your office?"*
- *"Who is the Veteran Experience Officer here?"*
- *"May I have the name and email of the Medical Center Director?"*

You'll learn how to use these names in escalation letters in later chapters.

Final Tip: You don't have to be rude to be effective. In fact, being calm, factual, and prepared is your best weapon.

Use phrases like:

- *"I'm asking for a resolution consistent with VHA Directive 1003."*
- *"I believe this warrants service recovery."*
- *"I'd like this documented in PATS, and I'd like a copy of the complaint."*

Sound informed. Sound reasonable. But never sound unsure.

Section 3 — When the Advocate Doesn't Do Their Job

If any of the following happen, you have grounds to escalate:

- They don't return your calls or secure messages
- They refuse to coordinate with clinical staff
- They fail to follow up
- They dismiss your concern without reviewing it

Don't argue. Just document it. Then go up the ladder. In Chapter 10, we'll show you how to write a formal complaint that cites their failure — with precision.

Section 4 — Quick Checklist: Working With a Patient Advocate

- ☐ Do you have a clear summary of what went wrong?
- ☐ Can you name the person or department responsible?
- ☐ Do you know what policy was likely violated?
- ☐ Are you making a specific request for correction?
- ☐ Did you request documentation in the PATS system?
- ☐ Are you prepared to escalate if ignored?

If you can check off these boxes, you're ready. If not, Chapters 4 and 6 will help you build the foundation.

Patient Advocates were created to help fix breakdowns in care. But that only works when you hold them to the role they were assigned — not the one they've grown comfortable with.

You don't have to beg for help. You have the right to expect advocacy. This chapter gave you the strategy. Chapter 7 will give you the law.

Next up: Learn how to use VA policy as a tactical tool to push the system toward action.

PART II

Advocacy in Action

> *"Knowing your rights is just the beginning. The real power comes when you start using them."*

This section moves from understanding the VA system to working within it strategically — on your terms.

Part II is about policy as power. Before you can challenge poor care or inaction, you need to know what the VA is actually required to do. Too many Veterans are shut down with vague excuses, stonewalled by bureaucracy, or told, *"That's just how it works."* But the truth is: VA staff have duties. VA programs have rules. And those rules are written down — in black and white.

These chapters will show you:

- How to turn VA directives into tools for getting care, services, and respect

- Which policies control the Veteran's experience, and how they apply to you

- What patient advocates are supposed to do — and what to do when they don't

The VA culture counts on Veterans never reading its internal rules. But once you do, you become harder to dismiss — and much harder to ignore. These aren't abstract regulations. They are leverage. And the sooner you start using them, the sooner you stop depending on luck, good moods, or the right staff being on duty.

If you've ever felt helpless in the system, this section will help you take that power back — one policy at a time.

Chapter 5: Using VA Policy to Strengthen Your Case

No Veteran enjoys filing complaints. It takes time, energy, and trust that someone will do something about it. But if you're reading this chapter, it likely means something has already gone wrong — and you've decided it's time to act.

This chapter shows you how to write complaints that cut through the noise and compel a response — not by ranting, but by using the VA's own rules. You'll learn how to cite policy, structure your message, and make sure it lands on the right desk with the right documentation. Done right, this becomes a powerful tool — not just for you, but for the next Veteran who walks through that door.

Section 1 — The Strategy Behind This Chapter

Most Veterans never see the VA's rulebook — let alone realize they can use it. But when care breaks down, written VA policy becomes your greatest tool. It's not about being aggressive. It's about being precise. When you point to a specific rule and ask why it wasn't followed, the conversation changes. Staff have to respond — not with opinion, but with action.

This chapter is your playbook for that moment.

You don't need to memorize regulations or quote obscure policy numbers from memory. What you need is a method. A plan. A way to recognize when VA staff are failing to follow their own guidance — and the confidence to do something about it.

Because here's the truth: VA staff are required to follow their own rules, even if they don't know them, don't agree with them, or are too busy to care. Your job isn't to argue. Your job is to point directly to the rule they're violating and ask one simple question:

"Can you show me where it says you're allowed to do that?"

In most cases, they can't — because the rule doesn't support what they're doing. And when you use VA policy as your foundation, you shift the burden. They now have to justify their behavior, not the other way around.

That moment became a turning point for me. I needed a private disability insurance form filled out — a policy I had from my job. The nurse told me that the doctor couldn't do it at the VA because VA policy would not allow it. When I asked the nurse if she could show me that policy, I was told to go home and find it myself. So I did. And what I found wasn't what she thought. And that moment was when the VA's rulebook stopped being their excuse — and started becoming my leverage.

What I found was VHA Directive 1134 — Completion of DBQs and Forms by VA Providers. This directive was very clear: VA doctors are required to fill out forms for Veterans — including private disability insurance paperwork, Social Security Disability function forms for your lawyer, and even Disability Benefits Questionnaires (DBQs). But more on that later.

Over the next several sections, you'll learn how to:

- Recognize when VA staff are out of compliance.
- Use federal law and VHA policy to challenge improper denials, delays, and excuses.
- Write effective complaints that force a written response.
- Escalate breakdowns to leadership — and trigger their accountability.

This chapter isn't about theory. It's about leverage. And it starts with knowing that the policy is already on your side.

Section 2 — Spotting When VA Isn't Following the Rules

One of the hardest parts of dealing with the VA system is recognizing when something is wrong — and knowing it's not your fault. When you don't get a call back, when referrals vanish into the void, when a nurse says, "*That's not our job,*" it's easy to second-guess yourself. But here's the truth: many of these breakdowns are not just bad service — they're violations of written VA policy.

This section will show you how to recognize those violations.

Start by asking yourself three questions:

1. Was I told something that doesn't sound right? For example:
   - "*We don't fill out those forms here.*"
   - "*You have to wait 30 days before we can act.*"
   - "*That's not how we do things at this facility.*"

If it sounds like a made-up rule, it probably is. That's your first red flag. And when you spot one, it's time to slow down, ask questions, and document what's happening

2. Did I get an answer with no explanation — or none at all?

    VA policy requires timely, transparent communication about decisions that affect your care. If you're left waiting without an answer or are told *"we're working on it"* indefinitely, that's a violation of VHA Directive 1003 — Veteran Patient Experience.

3. Was I denied access to care, information, or a service without being shown the rule that says I can't have it?

    VA employees don't get to make up restrictions on the spot. If they can't point you to a policy or law backing their decision, then their decision is likely out of compliance. This is where knowing even the name or number of a VHA Directive can shift the entire interaction.

Section 3 — Using VHA Policy to Push Back

You don't need to raise your voice to be powerful. When VA staff give you a runaround, policy gives you something stronger than emotion: authority.

Here's the core strategy: when you use the VA's own policies, you shift the conversation from "your opinion" versus "their opinion" to a question of compliance. VA staff can ignore frustration — but they can't ignore policy, especially when it's presented clearly and in writing.

Use These Three Steps:

Step 1 — Politely Ask for the Policy

When something doesn't feel right, trust that instinct. But instead of pushing back immediately, ask a simple, non-confrontational question:

"Can you show me the policy that supports what you're telling me?"

This does two things. First, it forces the staff member to consider whether they actually know the rule — or are just repeating what they've heard. Second, it gives them a chance to correct themselves without escalating the issue.

If they provide the policy, read it. If it supports your case, point it out. If they can't find it, you now have a strong reason to press further.

Step 2 — Find the Policy Yourself

If you're told no — especially without any policy citation — your next move is research. Many VA policies are publicly available on official websites. If you're dealing with care access, referrals, provider responsibilities, or complaint handling, you'll often find what you need in a VHA Directive or Handbook. At the time of writing this book, the link for all of the VHA Publications for the office and most current version was:

> https://www.va.gov/vhapublications/

If that link stops working in the future, Try searches like 'site:va.gov VHA Directive 1003.04' or 'DBQ form policy site:va.gov' to quickly find the official version.

If you are looking for a specific directive, you can reference Appendix A at the back of this guide — where I've listed the key policies Veterans use most often.

Step 3 — Use the Policy in Writing

Once you've found the policy, send it back to the VA — in a secure message or letter — and cite it directly. Keep it simple. Keep it professional. And always cite the policy directly:

> *"According to VHA Directive 1134, VA providers are required to complete private disability forms when medically appropriate. Please clarify why this was denied, and whether the provider has been informed of this requirement."*

This does two things: it puts your complaint into the record and forces VA staff to respond in writing — which becomes valuable evidence if you need to escalate later.

Section 4 — What to Do When They Ignore the Policy

Sometimes, even after you've clearly cited the correct VA policy, the system still doesn't budge. Staff brush you off. Phone calls aren't returned. You're told "we'll look into it," and then nothing happens. When that happens, you're not at a dead end — you're at a decision point.

Escalation isn't optional. It's part of the process.

VA policy isn't just for show — it's written with accountability mechanisms built in. When frontline staff fail to follow it, your next move is to escalate the issue to someone who's required to act. That includes Patient Advocates, clinic supervisors, service chiefs, and even Medical Center Directors. And when you're ignored at those levels, escalation continues up to the Veterans Integrated Service Network (VISN) Director and the Office of the Under Secretary for Health.

Start by restating the issue in writing:

- What happened
- Which policy was violated
- What you already tried to resolve it
- What you're asking them to do now

Keep your tone professional, not emotional — and always include a reference to the policy or directive they failed to follow. Don't just say you're frustrated. Show them the rule, and explain exactly how they broke it.

Use phrases like:

- "According to VHA Directive [####], VA staff are required to…"
- "This action contradicts VHA policy outlined in…"
- "Please provide a written explanation for this deviation from policy…"

These phrases don't just sound confident — they shift the legal and procedural burden back to the VA. Now they're the ones who must justify their actions. That's a very different conversation than simply pleading for help.

Chapter 5

When to escalate:

- If your secure messages or calls go unanswered
- If your Patient Advocate refuses to advocate
- If a service line ignores your documented complaint
- If the problem recurs despite prior attempts to fix it

Escalation isn't being difficult. It's doing exactly what VA policy expects a Veteran to do when the system isn't working. Escalating also creates a paper trail. And that matters — because when the next person reviews your case, that record becomes your strongest ally.

The next section will walk you through exactly how to write complaints that VA leadership can't ignore — and how to use your paper trail to your advantage.

Section 5 — Tracking and Documenting the Breakdown

When you're dealing with VA staff who aren't following policy, it's not enough to simply recall that you sent a few messages or made a couple of calls and expect the VA to take action. If you want to hold the system accountable, you have to create a record that shows what happened, what was supposed to happen, and how the system failed to meet its obligations. That's how you build leverage — and how you prepare for the next stage of advocacy.

Think of it this way: if you ever need to take your issue higher — to a Patient Advocate, a VISN Director, your Member of Congress, or the Office of Inspector General — they're going to ask for details. Being able to provide a clear, professional summary of events isn't just helpful — it makes you credible.

This kind of documentation becomes essential if you decide to involve external oversight like the Office of Inspector General (OIG), the Office of Resolution Management, Diversity & Inclusion (ORMDI), or even your Congressional representative. Each of these bodies will expect a factual, timeline-based summary of events supported by evidence. A well-kept log helps transform your concern from a personal grievance into a verifiable accountability issue — which is exactly what these oversight offices are designed to investigate.

This section will show you how to document the breakdowns in a way that supports your case and triggers accountability.

Start Your Own Complaint Log

A simple timeline or log of events can make all the difference. It doesn't have to be complicated. Just track four key things:

1. **Date** – When did it happen?
2. **Action** – What did you do (call, message, visit)?
3. **VA Response** – What did they say or do (or not do)?
4. **Policy Involved** – What policy or directive applies?

Sample Log Template (see Appendix E for more details):

Date	Action Taken	VA Response	Policy Involved	Next Step
Jan 5, 2025	Sent secure message requesting MRI results	No response	VHA Directive 1003	Follow-up msg, CC Patient Advocate
Jan 10, 2025	Called nurse triage line	Told "*they're backed up*"	VHA Directive 1003	Email summary to Mr. James; request written plan
Jan 12, 2025	Contacted Patient Advocate	Advocate said "*we just log complaints*"	38 U.S.C. § 7309A; VHA 1003.04	Escalate to Med Ctr Director if no reply by 25 Jan

Keep this log somewhere safe — and keep updating it. Every unanswered message or dismissive response builds your case.

Save the Evidence

Don't rely on memory. Keep records. This includes:

- Screenshots of secure messages and MyHealtheVet communication
- Copies of emails or faxes
- Notes from phone calls (date, time, who you spoke with)
- Appointment printouts or after-visit summaries

If something is said to you verbally — especially if it contradicts policy — write it down. Then follow up with a message confirming the conversation. For example:

> *"Just following up on today's phone call. You stated that VA providers are not allowed to complete private disability paperwork. I'd appreciate a written citation to the policy that supports that decision, or confirmation that this is being reviewed."*

Now the burden is on them to either back up the claim or walk it back.

Label Your Follow-Ups

As the problem drags on, make it clear that this is an unresolved issue — and that you're keeping track. You can do this professionally and effectively by labeling your messages clearly:

- Second Request – Unresolved Referral to Neurology
- Follow-Up – No Response from Patient Advocate
- Escalation to Service Chief – VHA Policy Violation
- Request for Written Explanation – VHA Directive 1003.04

This keeps your communication organized and signals that you're serious about pursuing resolution.

Use the Language of Accountability

VA policy uses words like "service recovery," "process improvement," and "complaint resolution." You can use those same terms when writing to staff or leadership:

- *"This matter appears to warrant **service recovery** under VHA Directive 1003."*
- *"This is a **recurring breakdown** and may reflect a larger **process failure**."*
- *"Please confirm whether this complaint has been **flagged for review** under your **Veteran Experience tracking** responsibilities."*

When you speak the VA's own language, you're no longer just a frustrated patient — you're a credible source pointing out a compliance failure that leadership has a duty to fix.

Chapter 5

Why It Matters

>Documenting the breakdown is not about keeping a personal journal. It's about building a professional, policy-based case that the system has failed — and giving leadership the opportunity (and the obligation) to correct it.

Because here's the truth: many problems at the VA don't get fixed the first time. But when a Veteran documents those failures in detail, cites the policies involved, and follows up persistently, those problems become harder to ignore — and impossible to dismiss.

Section 6 — Shifting Tactics: Building the Foundation for What Comes Next

By now, you've seen that VA policy isn't just background noise — it's a tool. When VA staff say, "*that's not how we do things*," policy is how you push back. When your care gets delayed or denied, policy gives you a foundation for action. When you're ignored, policy helps you escalate with confidence, not just frustration.

This chapter wasn't just about identifying problems — it was about learning to respond with precision, using the VA's own rules to make the system accountable to you.

And this is where everything else in this book starts to connect.

You've also laid the groundwork for credibility. Veterans who track their issues, cite policy, and document communication in writing are taken more seriously — not just by VA staff, but by oversight bodies and congressional offices. Your professionalism becomes part of your advocacy power.

In the chapters that follow, you'll learn how to take what you've built here — a clear understanding of VA's obligations — and apply it to some of the hardest parts of the system:

- When Patient Advocates refuse to advocate.
- When complaints get documented but not resolved.
- When supervisors and service lines go silent.
- When no one takes responsibility — and you're the one left without care.

You'll learn how to structure formal complaints, escalate them through the VA chain of command, and even trigger oversight reviews from outside watchdogs like the VA Office of Inspector General (OIG) or the Office of Resolution Management, Diversity & Inclusion (ORMDI). You'll also see how to protect your medical records — and challenge the VA when staff write false or misleading notes.

Everything from here forward builds on what you've just learned. Because once you know how to use VA policy to your advantage, you're not just another frustrated Veteran — you're someone who speaks the VA's language, cites its laws, and demands accountability on its own terms.

This is where the balance starts to shift. You now have tools the system can't ignore — and if they try, you'll know exactly where to escalate and how to make it matter. You're no longer waiting for the VA to do the right thing. You're holding them to it. And that changes everything.

Chapter 6: Applying Veteran Experience Policy to Your Situation

This chapter is a reference guide to the VA's customer service and experience policies — not just in theory, but as codified in federal law and internal VA directives. While Chapter 3 explained how these policies should affect your daily experience in the clinic, here we focus on the documents themselves: what they say, where they come from, and how to use them when the VA falls short.

Section 1 — 38 CFR § 0.601–0.603: The Legal Foundation for VA Culture

The Department of Veterans Affairs has legally adopted a set of core values and service standards in **Title 38, Code of Federal Regulations (CFR), Part 0**:

- **§ 0.601**: Establishes the "I CARE" values (Integrity, Commitment, Advocacy, Respect, Excellence)

- **§ 0.602**: Defines the six "Core Characteristics" of VA services (Trustworthy, Accessible, Quality, Innovative, Agile, Integrated)

- **§ 0.603**: Outlines the three pillars of customer experience: **Ease**, **Effectiveness**, and **Emotion**

These are not slogans. They are legally binding principles governing how VA employees are expected to treat Veterans, caregivers, and survivors in every interaction. If a VA employee dismisses your concern, speaks disrespectfully, or ignores your needs, you are experiencing a violation of these federal service standards.

These principles apply across every VA medical facility, community-based outpatient clinic, and Vet Center. They apply whether you are speaking to a receptionist, a scheduler, a nurse, or a specialist. VA culture is supposed to reflect these values — and when it doesn't, you have the right to call it out using the very standards VA claims to uphold.

Section 2 — The "I CARE" Values and What They Really Mean

The VA's official core values are:

- **Integrity**: Do what's right, even when no one is watching

- **Commitment**: Work diligently to serve Veterans and their families

- **Advocacy**: Identify and advance the interests of Veterans

- **Respect**: Treat all individuals with dignity

- **Excellence**: Strive for the highest quality in service

Of these, **Advocacy** is the most powerful for Veterans to invoke. The 38 CFR § 0.601 explicitly says:

"VA employees will be truly veteran-centric by identifying, fully considering, and appropriately advancing the interests of Veterans and other beneficiaries."

If you've ever been told "That's not my job" or "You need to talk to someone else," the staff member is likely ignoring this obligation. Every employee — not just those in advocacy roles — is required to proactively support Veterans.

When the VA fails to treat you with respect or simply ignores your request, you are not being difficult — you are being denied the basic standards built into VA's identity. This matters when you escalate, when you write a complaint, or when you prepare to contact Congress. You're not just expressing frustration — you're citing a failure to meet federally adopted policy.

Section 3 — CFR § 0.603: Customer Experience Standards That Must Be Met

Federal regulation § 0.603 defines the three essential components of all VA services:

- **Ease**: The process must be as simple and barrier-free as possible

- **Effectiveness**: Services must meet the Veteran's needs and provide the intended outcome

- **Emotion**: Veterans must feel respected, valued, and heard

These standards apply to:

- Phone calls
- Appointment scheduling
- Referrals and specialty access
- In-person and online interactions

Example:

> If you call repeatedly and no one returns your call, or if your specialty care referral disappears into a black hole, that is a violation of the "Ease" and "Effectiveness" standards. If you are treated rudely, dismissed, or ignored, that is a violation of the "Emotion" standard.

These aren't abstract concepts — they're legal expectations.

You don't have to quote these to a staff member at the front desk — but if you're being ignored or mistreated and later write a complaint to leadership or a Congressional office, citing CFR § 0.603 gives you more weight. It turns your complaint from "*I'm upset*" into "*This violates federal regulation.*"

Section 4 — VHA Directive 1003: Implementing the Veteran Experience Program

While The 38 CFR defines the overarching standards, VHA Directive 1003 puts them into action within the Veterans Health Administration. This directive mandates that:

- VA employees deliver care and service that reflects the "I CARE" values
- Every facility must implement a Veteran Patient Experience (VPE) program
- Service Recovery must be applied when breakdowns occur
- Veteran Experience Officers (PXOs) oversee implementation and improvement

Key provisions include:

- Use of "Own the Moment" and "VA Way" training for front-line staff
- Tracking and responding to complaints to improve systemic performance
- Evaluating staff and leadership based on their ability to meet experience standards

This directive is not a suggestion. It is a required operational standard for VA facilities and employees. If your local VA staff say, "There's nothing we can do," or "That's just how things work here," and leave the issue unresolved — they are violating this directive.

You can quote this directive directly in formal complaints or correspondence to show the VA is failing to meet its own mandated processes. Leadership cannot ignore these rules — they are accountable for ensuring they are followed.

Section 5 — Using These Policies to Strengthen Your Complaint or Appeal

If you are writing a complaint, appeal, or escalation letter, quoting policy increases credibility and impact. You can cite:

- **38 CFR § 0.603** to demonstrate failure to meet service standards
- **38 CFR § 0.601 (Advocacy)** when staff are indifferent to your concerns
- **VHA Directive 1003** when service recovery or corrective action is absent

Example language:

"*This experience violates CFR § 0.603, which requires that Veterans be treated with respect, ease of access, and effectiveness in service delivery.*"

"*Per VHA Directive 1003, VA employees are required to deliver care that reflects the agency's core values and to use service recovery when breakdowns occur. This has not been done.*"

Use this chapter as a reference when preparing:

- Formal complaints to Patient Advocates
- Written concerns to Medical Center Directors
- Escalations to VISN Directors or Congressional offices

When you make it clear that you understand these policies — and expect the VA to follow them — you change the conversation. You're no longer just another voice in the crowd. You're a Veteran holding them accountable to their own rules.

Section 6 — Summary: From Mission Statement to Binding Policy

- **CFR § 0.601**: Establishes VA's binding ethical values
- **CFR § 0.603**: Defines customer experience principles VA must meet
- **VHA Directive 1003**: Implements a nationwide program to enforce these principles and hold staff accountable
- These standards are legal, not optional — and staff failure to meet them can and should be documented
- Veterans can cite these standards in writing to demand respect, coordination, and corrective action

The VA often talks about "Whole Health" and "veteran-centered care," but this chapter proves that those aren't just ideals — they're obligations. The next time you're dismissed, delayed, or disrespected, don't just complain — cite the standard they failed to meet.

Next: The legal and policy framework that governs the Patient Advocacy Program itself.

Chapter 7: Understanding the Law Behind Patient Advocacy

This chapter is your formal reference guide to the Patient Advocacy Program. While Chapter 4 showed you how to work with Patient Advocates in practice, here we dive into the legal structure and policy framework that defines what the Patient Advocacy Program is *supposed* to be.

You'll learn:

- What federal law created the Patient Advocacy Program
- Which VHA directives govern how it operates
- What VA facilities and staff are required to do — and what they cannot ignore

When you understand this framework, you'll be equipped to challenge misinformation, demand accountability, and escalate your concerns with authority.

Section 1 — Federal Law: 38 U.S.C. § 7309A

The Patient Advocacy Program was created by Congress in 2016 under 38 U.S.C. § 7309A. This statute defines what the program must do, what Patient Advocates are responsible for, and how the entire system should function to protect the rights of Veterans. This law mandates that:

- Every VA medical center must have a Patient Advocacy Program
- Advocates must *advocate on behalf of Veterans* in health care matters
- Patient Advocates must understand the laws and rules related to Veterans' rights in VA health care

These are not suggestions — they are binding federal law.

Key clauses include:

- **§ 7309A(b)(1):** Establishes the Office of Patient Advocacy within the Veterans Health Administration.

- **§ 7309A(c)(2)(A):** "To advocate on behalf of Veterans with respect to health care received and sought by Veterans at the Department." Advocates must advocate for Veterans regarding VA health care.

- **§ 7309A(c)(2)(B):** Requires patient advocates to ensure Veterans understand their rights and responsibilities under VA care.

- **§ 7309A(d):** Details core responsibilities of Patient Advocates, including:
    - Receiving and documenting complaints
    - Educating Veterans about the complaint process
    - Coordinating with VA staff to address issues
    - Reporting complaint trends to improve care
    - Participating in training and evaluations
    - Required to know and understand the rules that govern VA health care, including federal law, VA regulations, and VHA directives.

These are statutory duties, meaning that VA employees and supervisors can be held accountable for noncompliance. When VA staff ignore these legal responsibilities, they are not simply making a mistake — they are violating the law.

38 U.S.C. § 7309A gives Veterans the foundation to demand more than a polite apology. It gives you the authority to demand action. This statute reinforces what every Veteran should expect from the Patient Advocacy Program: informed, accountable, and policy-driven support.

Section 2 — VHA Directive 1003.04: Patient Advocacy Program Policy

VHA Directive 1003.04 is the official VA policy document that explains how the Patient Advocacy Program must function. It applies to *every* VA medical center.

Key responsibilities from the directive:

- Document complaints in the Patient Advocate Tracking System (PATS)
- Coordinate with service lines until the issue is resolved
- Follow up and notify the Veteran of the outcome
- Collaborate with supervisors and Veteran Experience Officers (PXOs)
- Escalate system-wide issues to leadership

The directive also requires:

- Daily oversight by a Patient Advocate Supervisor
- Timely closure of complaints with full documentation
- Real-time data entry and tracking

Supervisors are expected to:

- Review unresolved complaints regularly
- Ensure proper documentation and closure in PATS
- Provide Just-in-Time (JIT) training to reinforce accountability

Patient Advocates cannot legally say:

- *"We just take notes."*
- *"That's not something I can help with."*
- *"We don't advocate anymore — we document."*

Those responses contradict both the directive and federal law.

VHA Directive 1003.04 requires Patient Advocates to take ownership of complaints. The policy states that Patient Advocates are responsible for *"addressing Veteran complaints at the point of service or referring the complaint to the appropriate staff for resolution while maintaining accountability for follow-up."* In other words, even if the solution lies with another department, the Advocate is still responsible for making sure it gets done.

VHA Directive 1003.04 also reinforces that every VA employee is expected to advocate for Veterans. The policy places this responsibility for training and ensuring staff meet this duty squarely on the Patient Advocate Supervisor.

Section 3 — The Oversight Structure

According to VA policy, the chain of accountability is built in:

- **Patient Advocates** must resolve or escalate complaints
- **Supervisors** must oversee the resolution and ensure compliance
- **Veteran Experience Officers (PXOs)** coordinate at the facility level
- **Medical Center Directors** are ultimately accountable for failures
- **VISN Directors** oversee multiple facilities and must intervene when systemic issues arise

This structure is designed for internal escalation. Use it.

The directive also mandates regular reporting and evaluation:

- Facilities must track recurring complaints
- Data must be used for quality improvement
- Complaint outcomes must be monitored by leadership teams

These requirements are not optional. They are conditions of VA health care governance.

Section 4 — When the System Fails: Using Policy in Your Complaint

If your Advocate fails to follow the rules, you should cite both:

- **38 U.S.C. § 7309A** (the law)
- **VHA Directive 1003.04** (the policy)

Examples:

> "Under 38 U.S.C. § 7309A(c)(2)(A), the Patient Advocate is required to advocate on my behalf regarding the health care issue I reported."

> "Per VHA Directive 1003.04, Patient Advocates are responsible for coordinating complaints until resolution and documenting outcomes in PATS. Neither occurred in this case."

Include this in escalation letters, complaints to facility directors, VISN leadership, or when contacting oversight bodies like the OIG or Congress.

Section 5 — Summary: Know the Law, Use the Policy

- Federal law *requires* VA Patient Advocates to advocate on behalf of Veterans
- VHA Directive 1003.04 defines how that advocacy must be carried out
- Complaints must be documented, resolved, and tracked in the PATS system
- Supervisors, PXOs, and Directors are all accountable for breakdowns
- If your Advocate fails to act, cite the law and policy directly when escalating

This chapter is your legal and procedural backbone. When strategy fails (see Chapter 4), structure wins. Use this framework to shift your complaint from frustration to enforcement.

> **Tip**: You can find the latest version of VHA Directive 1003.04 by searching: site:va.gov VHA Directive 1003.04 PDF

Next: Escalating beyond the facility — and getting results when local leadership fails.

Chapter 8: Responding When Patient Advocates Don't Help

The VA Patient Advocate is often described as your ally — someone who helps resolve problems, navigate systems, and ensure your concerns are heard. But what happens when they don't follow through, misrepresent your complaint, or simply forward your issue back to the very service line that failed you in the first place? This chapter explores what Patient Advocates are required to do under VA policy, how their role fits within the larger complaint system, and what options you have when they fail to act. Whether you're being ignored, dismissed, or gaslit, understanding the advocate's legal duties will help you respond with clarity and strength.

Here, you'll learn how to:

- Recognize when a Patient Advocate is out of compliance with their duties
- Respond effectively when they deflect, delay, or fail to act
- Elevate the issue with credibility and clarity
- Use their inaction as leverage in your broader case for accountability

The goal isn't to pick a fight. The goal is to restore function — to force a system that has stalled to take the action it was supposed to take in the first place. Because when Patient Advocates fail, they don't just fail you. They fail the next Veteran who walks through the door with the same problem.

Let's walk through what to do when the advocate doesn't advocate.

Section 1 — Recognizing When They Fail

It's not always obvious at first. You reach out to a Patient Advocate expecting help — and maybe you even get a polite response. But then nothing happens. Or what happens doesn't match what VA policy says should happen.

The reality is, not all Patient Advocates follow the law or the policies that define their role. Some may not be fully aware of what those responsibilities are. Others may be operating under local practices or internal pressures that keep them from fulfilling their full duties under VA policy. Regardless of the reason, the impact on the Veteran can be the same — unresolved issues and growing frustration.

This section will help you recognize when the Patient Advocate process isn't working the way it's supposed to — and how to distinguish between temporary delays and true breakdowns.

Watch For These Red Flags That a Patient Advocate May Not Be Meeting Their Responsibilities:

1. **They Only "Log" Your Complaint, But Don't Take Action**
   If you're told "we just document complaints and send them to the service line," that may indicate a misunderstanding of the advocate's actual role. Under VA policy, Patient Advocates are expected to actively facilitate problem resolution — not simply pass messages along.

   > **What VA Policy Says:** Under VHA Directive 1003.04 and 38 U.S.C. § 7309A, Patient Advocates must act as facilitators and problem-solvers — not passive messengers.

2. **They Defend the Department That Caused the Problem — Without Reviewing the Facts**
   If the Patient Advocate quickly sides with the service line or explains away the issue without taking time to understand your side or check the relevant policy, it may be a sign that they're not fulfilling their role as your advocate. Their responsibility is to investigate concerns, not automatically defend VA departments.

3. **They Seem Unfamiliar With Relevant Policy**
   If a Patient Advocate appears unaware of their responsibilities under VHA Directive 1003.04 or denies obligations without explanation, it may reflect gaps in training or local inconsistencies in how the role is defined. Veterans shouldn't assume this is intentional — but they also shouldn't ignore it.

4. **They Don't Communicate or Follow Through**
   Lack of follow-up — such as unanswered emails, missing updates, or unclear next steps — can quickly erode trust. This isn't always the result of negligence; some Patient Advocates may be overburdened. But regardless of the reason, timely communication is essential to the role.

5. **They Don't Flag Recurring Failures to Leadership**
   If multiple Veterans are experiencing the same issue — like repeated referral delays or misinformation — and it's not being escalated to leadership or quality management, that's a missed opportunity for systemic improvement. VHA policy explicitly expects Patient Advocates to track patterns and report them.

Why This Matters

When a Patient Advocate's support is limited — whether by training, staffing, or misunderstanding of their role — the breakdown doesn't just affect you. It leaves the next Veteran vulnerable to the same problem. That's why recognizing these warning signs matters — and why documenting them matters even more.

In the next section, you'll learn how to respond constructively when Patient Advocates fall short — including how to use policy, documentation, and professionalism to keep your case moving forward.

Section 2 — Common Excuses That Don't Hold Up

Patient Advocates should be allies in fixing care breakdowns. But when they fall short — whether from confusion, workload, or miscommunication — Veterans often hear explanations that simply aren't supported by policy. This section helps you recognize common excuses and respond with confidence, clarity, and citations.

Excuse #1: *"We just log complaints — we don't get involved."*

What to Know:
This is one of the most common — and most incorrect — statements Veterans hear. Patient Advocates are not passive scribes. They are required to act, not just record.

How to Respond:
"I understand your role includes logging complaints, but VHA Directive 1003.04 also requires you to actively help resolve issues and follow up with service lines. Can you clarify how that part is being handled in my case?"

Directive to Cite:
"Documenting Veteran complaints in PATS and coordinating resolution in partnership with SLAs. See paragraph 3.a. This includes ensuring the documentation entered is complete and actionable."
— **VHA Directive 1003.04(2)(I)(1)**

"Coordinating resolution for complaints that cannot be resolved at the point of service or require assistance from multiple service lines."
— **VHA Directive 1003.04(2)(I)(2)**

Chapter 8

"Providing guidance and support to SLAs in their efforts to address complaints in PATS, within their service line, by the designated timeframe."
— **VHA Directive 1003.04(2)(l)(4)**

Excuse #2: *"That's up to the clinic, not me."*

What to Know:
While clinical decisions belong to care teams, it's the Patient Advocate's duty to ensure the Veteran's concern is properly routed, tracked, and responded to — especially if care has been delayed or denied.

How to Respond:
"Under VHA Directive 1003.04, Patient Advocates are required to coordinate with clinics and service lines to help resolve access barriers. I'm not asking you to override the clinic — I'm asking you to help facilitate a proper response."

Directive to Cite:
"(2) Coordinating resolution for complaints that cannot be resolved at the point of service or require assistance from multiple service lines."
"(4) Providing guidance and support to SLAs in their efforts to address complaints in PATS, within their service line, by the designated timeframe."
— **VHA Directive 1003.04(2)(l)(2) & (4)**

"VHA patient advocacy utilizes PAs and SLAs across diverse services and departments who are dedicated to working with Veterans to address complaints that arise both at the point of service and when a complaint is received."
— **VHA Directive 1003.04(9)(d)**

Excuse #3: *"We don't advocate anymore — we're now called Customer Experience."*

What to Know:
This is a growing trend across some VA facilities, but a change in job title does not erase the legal obligations that remain in place. Patient Advocates are not a courtesy program — they are a legal requirement created by Congress to advocate on behalf of Veterans. Their core duties remain active, regardless of local rebranding efforts.

How to Respond:
*"While I understand local titles may differ, the law under 38 U.S.C. §

7309A still requires VA Patient Advocates to 'advocate on behalf of Veterans' with respect to health care. That responsibility hasn't changed."

Directive to Cite:
"(c)(2) *In carrying out the Patient Advocacy Program of the Department, the Director shall ensure that patient advocates of the Department — (A) advocate on behalf of Veterans with respect to health care received and sought by Veterans under the laws administered by the Secretary.*"
— **38 U.S.C. § 7309A(c)(2)(A)**

Excuse #4: *"You need to wait — we're still reviewing it."*

What to Know:
Timely communication is not optional. VHA Directive 1003 requires that Veterans be kept informed of delays or barriers affecting their care. "We're working on it" is not enough — updates must be timely and transparent.

How to Respond:
"*VHA policy requires that Veterans be given timely and meaningful updates about complaints and care access. Can you provide a specific timeframe or expected resolution date?*"

Directive to Cite:
"Taking corrective actions in a timely manner"
— **VHA Directive 1003(6)(c)(5)**

"(2)(i) *VA medical facility Service Chiefs are responsible for: (2) Providing oversight of complaints assigned to the service line in PATS and ensuring timely resolution based on designated timeframes and quality documentation that supports complaint closure.*"
— **VHA Directive 1003.04(2)(i)(2)**

"(2)(m) *The VA medical facility Organizational Specialist (FOS) is responsible for*: (3) *Ensuring ongoing communication with Veterans about their complaints, including pending actions and final resolution, until the complaint has been closed.*"
— **VHA Directive 1003.04(2)(m)(3)**

Excuse #5: *"We can't act unless the service line responds."*

What to Know:
Patient Advocates are not supposed to passively wait for the service line to act. They are responsible for **actively following up**, tracking unresolved concerns, and elevating them if needed.

How to Respond:
"VA policy requires Patient Advocates to follow up with the appropriate service lines and escalate when there's no timely response. I'm requesting that this issue be elevated to facility leadership or process improvement."

Directive to Cite:
"(2) Anticipating and correcting problems before they occur."
"(5) Taking corrective actions in a timely manner."
"(6) Ensuring appropriate follow-up and feedback to the Veteran."
— **VHA Directive 1003.04(c)(2) & (5) & (6)**

"(2) Coordinating resolution for complaints that cannot be resolved at the point of service or require assistance from multiple service lines."
"(3) Notifying the VA medical facility Patient Advocate Supervisor when very difficult or challenging complaints have been identified and more support is needed."
"(4) Providing guidance and support to SLAs in their efforts to address complaints in PATS, within their service line, by the designated timeframe."
— **VHA Directive 1003.04(2)(l)(2) & (3) & (4)**

Excuse #6: *"That's not my job — I don't handle clinical matters."*

What to Know:
Patient Advocates are not clinicians, but they are responsible for coordinating with clinical teams to help resolve concerns about access, communication, or breakdowns in care.

How to Respond:
"I'm not asking you to make a clinical decision. But per VA policy, you are required to coordinate with the service line when a Veteran raises a care-related concern."

Directive to Cite:
"(c)(2) In carrying out the Patient Advocacy Program of the Department, the Director shall ensure that patient advocates of the Department — (A) advocate on behalf of Veterans with respect to

Chapter 8

health care received *and sought by Veterans under the laws administered by the Secretary"*
— **38 U.S.C. § 7309A(c)(2)(A)**

"(2) Coordinating resolution for complaints that cannot be resolved at the point of service or require assistance from multiple service lines."
"(4) Providing guidance and support to SLAs in their efforts to address complaints in PATS, within their service line, by the designated timeframe."
— **VHA Directive 1003.04(2)(l)(2) & (4)**

Excuse #7: *"This has already been addressed — there's nothing more to do."*

What to Know:
Even if staff say the issue is *"closed,"* that doesn't mean it's been resolved correctly. If a Veteran is still experiencing the problem — or if the explanation was incomplete — the issue remains open under policy.

How to Respond:
"This issue has not been resolved from my perspective, and I'd like it reviewed again. VA policy allows for re-escalation when the Veteran remains dissatisfied or the issue recurs."

Directive to Cite:
"(n) VA medical facility Service Level Advocate are responsible for: (3) Assisting service lines in resolving issues after first attempts at resolution have not been successful and identifying opportunities for improvement within their service line or adjacencies with other service lines."
— **VHA Directive 1003.04(2)(n)(3)**

"Notifying the VA medical facility Patient Advocate Supervisor when very difficult or challenging complaints have been identified and more support is needed."
— **VHA Directive 1003.04(2)(l)(3)**

Excuses, no matter how common or confidently delivered, are not a substitute for policy. And now that you've seen how many of these common responses contradict VA's own rules, it's time to take the next step. In the next section, you'll learn how to use those same policies — the ones Patient Advocates are required to follow — to challenge inaction and force meaningful responses. It's not about confrontation. It's about precision. When you know the rules, you can hold the system to them.

Section 3 — Using Policy to Challenge Inaction

When you're getting nowhere — vague answers, delayed responses, or flat-out resistance — just like the common excuses we looked at in the last section, it's time to use something more powerful than frustration: **policy**.

The right response isn't to argue or plead. It's to point to the rules — the ones the VA is already required to follow. This section will show you how to use those policies to challenge inaction, keep the pressure on, and turn vague answers into documented responsibilities.

Policy-backed communication helps you stay focused, professional, and persistent — even when you're dealing with someone who isn't doing their job. Whether it's a Patient Advocate, service line staff, or even a facility leader, referencing the exact VA policy or federal statute forces them to take your concern more seriously.

Here's how to do it:

Step 1 – Ask for the Policy Politely
   If something doesn't sound right, don't argue — ask. Use respectful but clear language: *"Can you show me what VA policy supports that decision?"* *"Can you tell me what directive that's based on?"* This gives staff the opportunity to check their facts and may resolve the issue without conflict.

Step 2 – Cite the Policy Yourself
   If they don't offer a policy or if what they say doesn't match what you've read, respond with a clear reference to the appropriate directive or statute.

   Example: *"I reviewed VHA Directive 1003.04, and it says Patient Advocates are expected to coordinate resolution and follow up with service lines. Could you help me understand how that's being applied in my case?"*

Step 3 – Follow Up in Writing
   Always follow up in writing. Use MyHealtheVet secure messaging, email, or a written complaint form. Reference the policy and document the response (or lack of one). This creates a paper trail.

   Example: *"According to VHA Directive 1003.04, Paragraph 2(l)(2), Patient Advocates are responsible for coordinating resolution with service lines. I would appreciate clarification on who is currently handling this coordination."*

Step 4 – Escalate When Necessary

If no action is taken, escalate. State the policy again and explain that the current handling violates VA standards. Send your message to the next level up — the service line chief, facility director, or VISN contact. Keep your tone professional and reference the specific failure.

Example: *"I've raised this issue multiple times, and it remains unresolved. As outlined in VHA Directive 1003.04, the Patient Advocate is responsible for coordinating resolution and providing timely responses. I'm now requesting this issue be escalated to your supervisor or facility leadership."*

Being persistent, professional, and policy-based shifts the burden back to the VA — where it belongs. And when you document your concerns in writing, you're not just complaining — you're building a paper trail. That trail becomes critical if the issue still isn't resolved. In the next section, you'll learn how to escalate your concern in a way that demands a real response — not just another brush-off.

Section 4 — Writing an Escalation That Demands a Response

When policy-backed communication still doesn't get results, it's time to escalate — and how you write that escalation makes all the difference. A good escalation doesn't just vent frustration. It makes the problem impossible to ignore by outlining the facts, citing the policies, and showing exactly where VA staff failed to follow through.

In this section, you'll learn how to write an escalation that checks every box: it's professional, specific, well-documented, and backed by the VA's own rules. It shows that you've done your part — and that it's time for leadership to do theirs.

We'll cover:

- The core elements of a strong escalation message
- How to structure it step-by-step
- What tone to use (and avoid)
- How to attach your documentation and cite the right policy
- Where to send it — and how to follow up

This is where many Veterans feel stuck. But once you know how to put together a clear, policy-based escalation, the VA has fewer places to hide — and more pressure to respond.

Chapter 8

Escalating a problem doesn't mean being aggressive — it means being structured. Your goal is to write something that gets results, not just attention. That means creating a written escalation that shows:

- You've tried to resolve the issue already
- You understand the policies involved
- You're documenting the breakdown clearly
- You're requesting specific corrective action

Here's how to build that message:

Step 1 – Start with a Brief Summary of the Problem

Be specific, but concise. Don't recount every detail — just summarize the key failure.

Example:

"I'm writing to follow up on an unresolved referral to Neurology that was requested on May 5. Despite multiple inquiries, I have not received a response or appointment. This delay has negatively affected my care."

Step 2 – Show That You Tried to Resolve It

Mention your past attempts — calls, messages, or visits — and what the result (or lack thereof) was.

Example:

"I sent two MyHealtheVet messages (May 10 and May 17), called the Nurse Triage line (May 19), and spoke to a Patient Advocate (May 22), but the issue remains unresolved."

Step 3 – Cite the Policy That Applies

This is where you shift the conversation from frustration to accountability. Use the policy language to define the failure.

Example:

"Under VHA Directive 1003.04, Patient Advocates are required to coordinate resolution of complaints and ensure they are addressed within designated timeframes. This has not occurred in my case."

Chapter 8

Step 4 – State What You're Asking For

Be direct. What action are you requesting?

Example:

"I am requesting that this referral be reviewed immediately and that I receive a response confirming the current status and next steps."

Step 5 – Make It Easy to Respond

Close with a polite, professional invitation to respond — and make clear you're tracking the timeline.

Example:

"Please respond by [date] so I can determine whether additional steps are necessary. Thank you for your attention to this matter."

Putting It All Together: Sample Escalation Message

Subject: Escalation – Unresolved Neurology Referral

I'm writing to follow up on an unresolved referral to Neurology that was submitted on May 5. I've sent secure messages on May 10 and May 17, called the Nurse Triage line on May 19, and spoke with a Patient Advocate on May 22. However, the referral remains pending, and I have not received a timeline or response.

Under VHA Directive 1003.04, Patient Advocates are responsible for coordinating resolution and ensuring timely updates. That has not occurred in this case.

I respectfully request that this issue be reviewed by the appropriate service line, and that I receive a written update regarding next steps no later than [insert date].

Thank you for your assistance.

Next Step:

By now, you've likely taken your concern as far as the Patient Advocate Supervisor. But if the issue still isn't resolved, it's time to go higher. Chapter 9 will walk you through how to escalate your complaint beyond the local level — to senior medical center leadership, VISN officials, the VA Office of Inspector General, or even your Member of Congress.

Section 5 — When and How to Involve Leadership and VISN

If you've cited policy, followed up in writing, and even escalated to the Patient Advocate Supervisor — but your concern is still unresolved — it's time to take your issue higher. VA leadership is responsible for ensuring their teams follow the law and uphold the standards set by VA directives. And when internal accountability breaks down, regional and national oversight structures exist to intervene.

This section will show you how and when to raise your concerns to medical center leadership and your facility's regional network: the Veterans Integrated Service Network (VISN).

When to Escalate Beyond the Facility

Not every delay or disagreement needs to go to the top. But here are clear signs that leadership-level escalation is appropriate:

- You've submitted multiple complaints but received no action or meaningful response.

- The Patient Advocate or their supervisor is ignoring documented VA policy.

- A service line is stonewalling or refusing to address a recurring problem.

- You suspect broader systemic failures that affect other Veterans, not just yourself.

- You've been told "there's nothing more we can do" despite clear obligations under policy.

If any of these apply, escalation isn't just appropriate — it's necessary.

Who to Contact

Depending on the situation, you may escalate to one or more of the following:

1. **Veterans Experience Officer (VEO)**
   Most VA Medical Centers have a designated VEO responsible for overseeing the entire patient experience program, including how complaints are handled. Some report directly to the Director.

2. **Medical Facility Director**
   These are the senior officials at your VA facility. You can address a formal letter or email to the Director's Office, clearly stating that the issue was not resolved through the Patient Advocate process.

3. **VISN Leadership**
   Each VISN oversees multiple VA facilities in a region. They provide oversight and enforce consistency across hospitals and clinics. You can submit complaints to the VISN Director or VISN-level Veterans Experience Program office.

4. **VA Office of Inspector General (OIG)**
   If you believe there is misconduct, gross mismanagement, falsified records, or systemic failure, the VA OIG has jurisdiction to investigate. Their online form accepts detailed complaints with supporting evidence.

How to Write an Effective Leadership-Level Escalation

The same principles apply: keep it professional, cite policy, and document everything. But at this level, your tone should emphasize the systemic nature of the failure and the lack of internal resolution.

Include:

- A clear timeline of what you did and when.
- What policy was violated or ignored.
- The impact on your care or rights.
- What resolution you're seeking.
- Any attachments (logs, messages, directives).

Sample opening:

"I am writing to formally request leadership review of a complaint that has not been resolved through the local Patient Advocacy process. Despite multiple follow-ups, the response I've received contradicts the responsibilities outlined in VHA Directive 1003.04 and 38 U.S.C. § 7309A..."

Keep a copy of everything you send and log your escalation as part of your ongoing documentation.

Why It Works

Patient Advocates are supposed to be the safeguard — the ones who step in when the system fails. But too often, they become another layer of delay, deflection, or silence. This chapter gave you the tools to understand their duties and how to hold them to them. You now know what they're supposed to do, what they're not allowed to ignore, and how to respond when they fail.

You don't need anyone's permission to speak up. And if the Patient Advocate won't help — that's not the end of your complaint. It's the beginning of your escalation.

The next step is writing a complaint that sticks — one that leadership and oversight bodies can't ignore.

PART III

Escalation and Enforcement

> *"When the system doesn't listen, you go up the chain — and you bring documentation with you."*

Sometimes understanding the system and quoting policy isn't enough. You follow the rules. You file a complaint. You ask for help. And nothing happens. That's when it's time to escalate.

This section is about what to do when your care hits a wall — when internal advocates fail, leadership deflects, and VA policy is ignored. It will show you how to push forward using the tools VA can't block: the chain of command, Congressional oversight, and the VA Office of Inspector General (OIG).

You'll also learn:

- How to write complaints that get attention and are hard to dismiss
- How to avoid common mistakes that weaken your case
- Why persistence — with documentation — is your greatest asset

You don't need to be a lawyer to hold the VA accountable. But you do need a strategy. These chapters will walk you through the escalation playbook — so that when you hit resistance, you don't stop. You escalate smart, and you escalate strong.

The system may not want to be held accountable — but it has no choice when you know how to make your voice heard.

Chapter 9: Escalating Complaints Beyond the Local VA

At some point, many Veterans find themselves stuck in a loop — delays with no answers, staff who stop responding, and a Patient Advocate who logs the complaint but never follows up. When this happens, it's time to step beyond the local facility.

This chapter is about escalation — not out of anger, but out of necessity. When local efforts fail, VA's own structure offers a pathway upward: from the Medical Center Director, to the Veterans Integrated Service Network (VISN), to national offices in Washington, D.C. And if that isn't enough, Congress and the VA Office of Inspector General (OIG) each offer oversight tools that can bring powerful scrutiny to unresolved issues.

But escalation only works if you know how — and when — to do it.

This chapter will give you a clear map of the chain of command and oversight process, explain what each level is responsible for, and help you determine the right audience for your complaint. You'll also learn what Congress can (and can't) do to help you, what the OIG investigates, and how to avoid wasting time on routes that won't lead anywhere.

If you've built a strong foundation — documented the breakdowns, cited the right policies, and followed up professionally — this is where that work begins to pay off.

Section 1 — The Chain of Command: Medical Center to VISN to VA Central Office

If your concerns haven't been resolved at the Patient Advocate or service line level, the next step is to follow the VA's own internal chain of command. VA health care is structured in tiers — and each level has oversight responsibility for the level below it. When used correctly, this structure gives you a clear and legitimate path for escalating unresolved problems.

Step 1: The Medical Center Director

> Every VA Medical Center (VAMC) has a Director who serves as the senior executive for the entire facility. That person is ultimately responsible for ensuring that care is delivered in accordance with VA policy and that staff are held accountable for failures.

If your complaint involves delayed care, unanswered messages, or breakdowns in patient advocacy, and those issues remain unresolved despite your efforts, you have the right to escalate directly to the Medical Center Director. Your escalation should be:

- **Professional** — Stick to the facts and focus on the policy failures.

- **Documented** — Include a timeline, past efforts to resolve the issue, and relevant policy citations.

- **Targeted** — Ask for specific corrective actions or follow-up.

Tip: You can usually find the Medical Center Director's name and office contact on the VAMC's official website under "Leadership."

Step 2: VISN Leadership (Regional Oversight)

If the Medical Center Director does not respond or fails to resolve the problem, the next level up is the VISN — the Veterans Integrated Service Network. VA health care is divided into 18 VISNs across the country. Each VISN oversees multiple VA Medical Centers and is responsible for ensuring that facilities within its network comply with national standards.

Each VISN has a Network Director (the senior executive), and a Veteran Experience Officer or equivalent who handles escalated patient care concerns. At this level, your message should:

- Clearly state that you are escalating due to unresolved issues at the facility level.

- Include all prior correspondence or a summary of efforts made.

- Emphasize that you are requesting regional oversight under VA policy and customer service standards.

Tip: VISN Public Affairs or Veteran Experience email addresses are usually listed on the VA's VISN directory.

Step 3: VA Central Office (National Leadership)

If both the Medical Center and VISN have failed to address the issue, you can escalate to VA Central Office (VACO) in Washington, D.C. While responses at this level can vary, it serves as a final

Chapter 9 56

administrative escalation route within the VA before involving oversight bodies like Congress or the OIG.

Key offices within VACO that may receive escalations include:

- The **Under Secretary for Health** (through public affairs or policy channels)

- The Office of the Deputy Under Secretary for Health for Operations

- The Veteran Experience Office (VEO) at the national level

Your escalation should be concise but thorough. Focus on the failure of the previous levels to correct the issue, and cite not only facility-level failures but also VISN inaction, if applicable. Keep a professional tone and request specific follow-up or accountability under applicable laws and directives.

Escalating through the chain of command ensures that your complaint follows the same accountability structure VA is supposed to use internally. When you present a clear paper trail and reference the right directives, you signal that you understand the system — and expect it to function as designed.

Section 2 — When to Use Congressional Assistance

Every Veteran has the right to request help from their elected representatives in Congress. While Congress doesn't manage the day-to-day operations of the VA, each U.S. Senator and House Representative has staff specifically assigned to help constituents navigate federal agencies — including the VA. These are often called **congressional liaisons** or **veteran caseworkers**, and their job is to intervene when the system isn't working the way it should.

But timing matters. Congressional offices can be a powerful tool — when used strategically.

Knowing when to involve your Member of Congress depends not only on how many steps you've taken within the VA system, but also on the seriousness of the issue — especially if your health or safety is at risk. In general, it's best to give the VA a reasonable opportunity to respond, usually between 14 to 30 days. Make a good-faith effort to resolve the problem by working first with the Patient Advocate, then escalating to Medical Center leadership if needed. If those channels don't produce results, taking your concern to the Veterans Integrated Service Network (VISN) is the usual next step.

However, when delays could result in serious health consequences, it may be appropriate to contact your congressional representative earlier — even as soon as your case reaches the Patient Advocate Supervisor level. In urgent situations, early congressional intervention can help break through bureaucratic barriers and prompt a faster response.

Once you've created a clear paper trail and the VA has either failed to act or taken action that places you at risk, congressional help becomes a legitimate next step. Intervention is most effective when all reasonable efforts to resolve the matter within the VA have been exhausted — or when those efforts are clearly failing. This includes situations where medically necessary care is delayed or denied, policies are ignored, or formal complaints go unanswered or are prematurely closed without resolution.

Congressional support is also appropriate if you've faced retaliation for raising concerns, or if you believe your rights have been violated and internal oversight — including the Patient Advocate or VISN leadership — has not taken corrective action. In these cases, your Member of Congress can bring additional visibility and accountability to your situation and help ensure that your voice is not ignored.

What a Congressional Office Can Do

Congressional staff have several tools available to assist Veterans who are experiencing problems with the VA. Congressional staff can:

- Submit a formal inquiry to the VA on your behalf.
- Ask for an expedited response or resolution.
- Require the VA to explain why certain decisions were made.
- Elevate your concern to national VA leadership or oversight offices.
- Track your case and follow up if the VA does not respond.

These inquiries often get attention quickly — especially when your communication is professional, policy-based, and well-documented.

What a Congressional Office Cannot Do

Congressional offices cannot:

- Force the VA to grant disability compensation or increase a rating.
- Override clinical medical decisions or substitute their judgment for a provider's.
- Replace the formal appeal process for VA benefits decisions.
- Guarantee a specific outcome.

Congressional staff can help you get clear answers, enforce response deadlines, and expose policy violations. But they can't rewrite federal regulations or pressure individual providers to make a certain call.

How to Make a Strong Congressional Request

To be effective, your request for congressional assistance should:

- Be concise — usually one page or less. Let the supporting documents provide the details.
- Summarize what happened, what should have happened, and what went wrong.
- List your attempts to resolve the issue within the VA.
- Cite relevant VA policies or federal law.
- Attach supporting documentation (letters sent or received, secure messages, complaint logs, denials, etc.).
- Be respectful — assume the congressional office wants to help, and give them a clear path to do so.

You can send your request via email, online case form, or physical mail. Many congressional offices now have online submission portals specifically for VA issues.

Congressional intervention isn't just about making noise — it's about restoring accountability. When the internal VA process breaks down, your Member of Congress can step in as an external check, demanding answers the VA might otherwise avoid.

Used wisely, congressional help can break logjams and restore access to the care and respect you deserve.

Section 3 — What the OIG Investigates (and What They Don't)

When internal VA channels fail — or when serious misconduct is involved — the VA Office of Inspector General (OIG) becomes a powerful oversight tool. But it's important to know what the OIG does (and does not) investigate, so your complaint is properly directed and has the best chance of being accepted.

The VA OIG is an independent agency tasked with investigating serious problems involving waste, fraud, abuse, gross mismanagement, or violations of law within the Department of Veterans Affairs. That includes failures in health care delivery, but only under certain conditions. The OIG is not a general complaint line or a customer service center.

Your complaint must involve more than a frustrating experience or a single rude staff member. It must raise legitimate concerns about systemic failure, risk to patient safety, repeated negligence, or illegal conduct.

Common Types of Complaints OIG May Accept

- Patient harm caused by delays, neglect, or improper care
- Falsified or misleading medical records
- Failure to follow mandatory policies or procedures
- Abuse of authority, whistleblower retaliation, or ethics violations
- Unlawful denial of care, access, or benefits
- Widespread issues in the operation of a VA clinic or medical center
- Misuse of VA funds or government resources

What the OIG Typically Doesn't Investigate

- Personality conflicts or isolated staff rudeness
- Billing disputes or travel pay complaints
- Disagreements over medical judgment when proper procedures were followed
- Requests to change or override disability compensation decisions (those go through the Veterans Benefits Administration or Board of Veterans' Appeals)
- Complaints already being handled appropriately at the facility or VISN level

Strategic Tip: If your issue involves a policy violation or a facility's failure to follow internal procedures, try exhausting the chain of command first — including the Patient Advocate Supervisor and VISN leadership. The OIG will want to know what steps you've taken before reaching out to them.

But if you believe you are facing **serious harm, ongoing safety risks,** or **retaliation for speaking up,** you do not need to wait. The OIG accepts direct complaints from Veterans and may intervene if the issue meets their criteria

Section 4 — How to File an Effective Complaint with the OIG

Filing a complaint with the VA Office of Inspector General (OIG) is a serious step — and when done correctly, it can trigger oversight, investigations, and even systemic reform. But to be effective, your complaint must be clear, credible, and focused on the kinds of issues the OIG is empowered to investigate.

What to Include in Your Complaint

A strong OIG complaint should answer three core questions:

1. **What happened?**
   Describe the incident(s) clearly and factually. Stick to the timeline. Be specific about dates, locations, and the names or titles of VA staff involved.

2. **Why is this serious?**
   Explain why this is not a simple misunderstanding or isolated incident. Focus on policy violations, gross mismanagement, patient safety issues, or legal misconduct.

3. **What evidence do you have?**
   Reference emails, medical records, documented conversations, or other proof. Avoid overwhelming the complaint letter itself with attachments. Instead, organize your supporting material into clearly labeled **appendices**.

Use Appendices to Keep It Focused and Professional

An effective way to structure your OIG submission is to use **appendices** to hold the details — so your main complaint remains short, direct, and well-documented.

Why Use Appendices?

- Keeps your complaint letter focused and readable.
- Allows you to present timelines, policy citations, emails, and exhibits in a clean, organized format.
- Shows professionalism and structure — which builds credibility.

Tips for Organizing Your Appendices:

- Use separate labels: Appendix A – Timeline of Events, Appendix B – Secure Message Screenshots, Appendix C – Policy Citations, etc.
- Clearly reference each appendix from within the main complaint:
  "As detailed in Appendix A, this delay spanned more than 30 days with no response despite multiple follow-ups."
- Number your exhibits within each appendix for easy cross-referencing:
  "See Appendix B, Exhibit 3 – Secure message dated March 14, 2025."

Example Appendix Structure:

- Appendix A – Chronology of Events
- Appendix B – Evidence of Communication Attempts
- Appendix C – Relevant Policy or Directive Excerpts
- Appendix D – Summary of Previous Escalation Efforts
- Appendix E – Supporting Medical Notes or Impacts

This structure allows you to say more by writing less — presenting a professionally prepared complaint that gives the OIG everything they need, without overwhelming them with disorganized information.

Example Phrases That Strengthen Your Complaint

- *"This appears to violate VHA Directive [number], which requires..."*
- *"This delay in care has resulted in worsening symptoms and could lead to serious harm."*
- *"Despite escalating through the appropriate chain of command, no action has been taken."*
- *"This appears to reflect a pattern of systemic failure at [facility name]."*

Where to File

You can submit a complaint to the VA OIG through:

- **Online:** https://www.va.gov/oig/hotline/default.asp
- **Phone:** 800-488-8244
- **Fax:** 202-495-5861
- **Mail:**
  VA Inspector General Hotline (53H)
  810 Vermont Avenue, NW
  Washington, D.C. 20420

What Happens After You File

- You may receive a confirmation, but you won't always be updated on the outcome.
- If the OIG accepts the complaint, they may launch a formal investigation or refer it to another oversight body within the VA.
- If the issue is better handled at a lower level, the OIG may forward it to the facility or VISN — which is why having already tried those steps strengthens your complaint.

Final Tip: Treat your OIG complaint like a legal brief — concise, factual, and supported with properly referenced appendices. Avoid venting or emotional language. Your goal is to demonstrate a pattern of mismanagement, misconduct, or serious risk — and provide the OIG with the organized documentation they need to take action.

But a strong complaint is just the beginning. What you do next — how you follow up and maintain pressure — will often determine the outcome.

Chapter 10: Writing Complaints That Get Attention

When the VA fails to follow its own policies, the most powerful response you can make is a well-documented, policy-backed complaint. These aren't just angry letters — they are legal and administrative tools that compel the VA to respond. Whether you're writing to a Patient Advocate, Service Line Chief, Facility Director, or even Congress, how you present your complaint can determine whether it's ignored or escalated. This chapter breaks down how to structure your complaints, what language to use, how to cite relevant policies, and how to build a paper trail that leaves no room for deflection. When done right, your words become leverage.

In the pages ahead, you'll learn:

- How to tailor your message to the audience,
- How to center your complaint around specific policy failures,
- How to structure it step-by-step for clarity and impact,
- And how to organize and reference supporting evidence in appendices.

By the end of this chapter, you'll have the tools to write a complaint that commands attention, withstands bureaucratic deflection, and triggers real accountability.

Let's start by understanding exactly who is reading what you write — and why that matters.

Section 1 — Know the Audience: Who Reads What You Write

Writing an effective complaint starts with knowing who will read it — because how you write it should depend on where it's going. A message sent to a Patient Advocate Supervisor should sound different from one sent to VISN leadership or a Member of Congress. Understanding your audience — and the scope of their authority — helps you strike the right tone, cite the right policies, and include the right level of detail.

Complaint to a Patient Advocate Supervisor

Primary Purpose: Internal resolution and Patient Advocacy program accountability

Audience Role: Oversees the patient advocacy team and day-to-day complaint handling

Tone to Use: Firm but cooperative

What to Include:

- Reference to specific policy (especially VHA Directive 1003.04)
- Summary of failed efforts to resolve with front-line advocates
- A clear, policy-based request for corrective action
- Indication you're trying to resolve this before further escalation

Example:
"I'm requesting a formal review of how my complaint was handled by the Patient Advocate Office. Under VHA Directive 1003.04, certain follow-up actions are required but were not taken. Please advise how this will be addressed and documented in PATS."

Complaint to the Patient Experience Officer (If Your Facility Has One)

Primary Purpose: Address broader trends or breakdowns in the patient experience

Audience Role: Senior official tasked with improving Veteran experience and often supervising the Patient Advocate Supervisor

Tone to Use: Professional and focused on systemic concerns

What to Include:

- Persistent patterns or failures in Veteran treatment
- Lack of responsiveness from the Patient Advocate team
- Cited policies (especially those in VHA Directives 1003 and 1003.04)
- A request for intervention or clarification of how complaints are being handled

Example:
"I am writing to bring your attention to repeated failures by the Patient Advocacy Office to follow basic responsibilities under VHA Directive 1003.04. These breakdowns appear to reflect larger issues in the facility's approach to Veteran experience."

Complaint to the Medical Center Director

Primary Purpose: Leadership accountability when internal mechanisms fail

Audience Role: Top official responsible for all operations at the medical facility

Tone to Use: Direct and fact-driven

What to Include:

- Failed attempts to resolve through Patient Advocacy or Patient Experience Officer
- Summary of the breakdown, including relevant dates and policy references
- Concise statement of harm or risk caused by inaction
- A request for personal review or redirection

Example:
"This issue remains unresolved despite multiple attempts to seek resolution through the appropriate VA channels. I am now requesting your direct oversight, as this involves potential violations of VHA Directive 1003.04 and impacts continuity of care."

Complaint to VISN Leadership

Primary Purpose: Oversight beyond the local medical center

Audience Role: Regional authority supervising multiple VA medical centers

Tone to Use: Formal, concise, and documentation-heavy

What to Include:

- Summary of failures at the facility level, including nonresponse by director
- Clear citations of breached VA directives
- Attachments with evidence or a structured appendix
- A specific request for regional review and facility-level accountability

Example:
"Due to lack of corrective action at the facility level, I am requesting that VISN 08 leadership review this matter. Attached is a summary of policy violations and communication history with the Fort Myers VA Clinic."

Complaint Sent Through a Congressional Office

Primary Purpose: Trigger external oversight and escalate unresolved or serious concerns

Audience Role: Congressional staff acting as liaisons to VA leadership

Tone to Use: Respectful, factual, and documentation-backed

What to Include:

- A brief and clear summary of the issue in plain language
- Supporting documentation and referenced VA policies
- Evidence of failed internal escalation attempts
- A statement of risk or serious concern (e.g., delayed care, policy violations, retaliation)

Example:
"I am asking for your office's help with a care delay at the Fort Myers VA Clinic. Multiple attempts to resolve this through the facility have failed, despite clear VA policy requiring timely follow-up. Attached is a timeline and documentation."

Quick Reference Table: Choosing the Right Complaint Strategy

Complaint Target	Primary Purpose	Tone to Use	What to Include
Patient Advocate Supervisor	Address poor handling of a complaint by front-line PAs	Firm but cooperative	Cite VHA Directive 1003.04; describe unresolved issue; request corrective action
Patient Experience Officer	Address systemic or repeated breakdowns in Veteran care	Professional and focused	Highlight patterns; cite VHA Directives 1003 & 1003.04; request oversight or intervention
Medical Center Director	Demand accountability from facility leadership	Direct and fact-driven	Summarize failed steps; reference policy violations; state harm or ongoing risk
VISN Leadership	Escalate above local facility for regional intervention	Formal and concise	Outline unresolved issues; cite relevant directives; include attachments or appendix
Congressional Office	External oversight for serious or unaddressed concerns	Respectful and clear	Provide plain-language summary; show failed attempts to resolve; attach policy-based evidence

Section 2 — Building a Complaint with Policy at Its Core

Every strong VA complaint has two parts: your experience and the policy that was violated. It's not enough to just say what went wrong — you need to explain why it was wrong according to the VA's own rules.

That's what turns a complaint into something leadership must answer, not just acknowledge.

When you connect your experience to a specific policy or federal regulation, you're no longer just reporting a bad outcome. You're documenting noncompliance. That changes how your complaint is viewed and how seriously it must be taken.

Chapter 10

Many Veterans assume that when they go to the Patient Advocate's office, their complaint will be reviewed according to VA policy — that the rules will be understood and applied. But in reality, many complaints are handled based on local habits or incomplete understanding. Complaints that clearly connect the issue to written policy are more likely to be taken seriously and acted upon.

That's why learning how to cite the right policies — and use them strategically in your complaint — is one of the most powerful tools a Veteran can develop.

Complaints grounded in policy do three things:

1. **They clarify the problem.** Instead of a vague frustration, the issue becomes a clear violation of a known rule.

2. **They force accountability.** When you cite the regulation, it puts the burden back on the VA to explain why their actions don't match what the rules require.

3. **They raise the stakes.** Policy violations often require involvement from higher-level leadership, compliance officers, or even external oversight bodies.

To build this kind of complaint, you need more than a personal account — you need a clear structure that connects your experience to the policy breakdown. The following five steps will help you organize your complaint in a way that is professional, persuasive, and grounded in VA rules.

Step 1: Identify What Went Wrong

Start by clearly stating the problem. What was the service failure, delay, or denial? Be specific about what you expected to happen and what actually happened.

Example:

"I requested follow-up on my neurology referral, but despite multiple inquiries over the last four weeks, I have received no communication from my care team."

Step 2: Link It to a Policy or Law

Use VA policies, directives, or federal statutes to frame why the issue matters. You can refer back to earlier chapters, or the Policy Reference Tables at the back of this book.

Example:

"According to VHA Directive 1003.04, Patient Advocates are required to coordinate complaint resolution with the responsible service lines and provide prompt and thorough responses (Paragraph 2(l)(2)-(3))."

Step 3: Be Professional and Direct

The tone of your complaint matters. Be firm but respectful. You're not venting — you're documenting. Keep emotions in check and use language that signals seriousness.

Example:

"I am requesting that this complaint be formally reviewed and responded to in accordance with VHA Directive 1003.04. Please advise who is currently handling this matter and what steps are being taken."

Step 4: Add Any Supporting Evidence

If you have notes, screenshots, appointment records, or messages that support your case, briefly refer to them and attach them separately. If the complaint will be long, include the evidence in an appendix and label it clearly.

Example:

See Appendix A for a timeline of contacts and communication attempts.

Step 5: State What You Want

Be clear about the resolution you're seeking — whether it's a referral, an explanation, or a corrective action.

Example:

"I am requesting an immediate update on the status of my neurology referral and a response to why no communication has been provided since the original request."

Checklist: Building a Complaint with Policy at Its Core

Before You Write:

- ☐ Identify what went wrong — the experience you want to report.
- ☐ Determine which policy, directive, or regulation was violated.
- ☐ Make sure you can clearly explain **why** it was wrong based on VA rules.

Use These Tips to Strengthen Your Complaint:

- ☐ Keep your tone respectful, direct, and professional.
- ☐ Stay fact-based. Avoid speculation or emotional exaggeration.
- ☐ Be specific — include names, dates, and the service or department involved.
- ☐ Use quotes or paraphrased text from the relevant VA policy when possible.

Sources You Might Reference:

- ☐ VHA Directives (e.g., 1003.04 for Patient Advocacy, 1110.02 for Social Work)
- ☐ 38 U.S.C. § 7309A (Federal law on Patient Advocacy)
- ☐ CFR § 0.603 (Customer Experience Standards)

Section 3 — Structuring Your Complaint: Step-by-Step Guide

Once you've identified the problem and linked it to policy, the next step is to present it in a way that's clear, concise, and professional. A well-structured complaint isn't just easier to read — it makes it harder for VA staff to dismiss or deflect. When your complaint flows logically and stays grounded in VA policy, it forces attention, invites accountability, and increases the odds of a meaningful resolution.

Veterans often wonder what kind of complaint will actually lead to change. Through years of advocacy experience and real-world use, a clear pattern has emerged: the most effective complaints follow a structured approach grounded in policy, facts, and clarity. This structure isn't just intuitive — it mirrors the same format used in legal, administrative, and congressional settings, and it aligns with how the VA expects complaints to be presented under its own policies. When your complaint is built this way, it's more likely to be understood, taken seriously, and acted upon by those in a position to fix the problem.

Below is a proven structure for writing complaints that get taken seriously.

1. Opening Paragraph: Who You Are and Why You're Writing

Start with a short paragraph that introduces who you are, your status as a Veteran enrolled in VA care, and why you are submitting a formal complaint.

Example:

> "My name is John Smith, and I am a service-connected Veteran currently enrolled in care at the Bay Pines VA Medical Center. I am writing to submit a formal complaint regarding delayed access to care that I believe violates established VA policy and has resulted in unnecessary risk to my health."

2. Background: What Happened and When

Briefly outline the key facts and timeline. Keep it focused and objective. If needed, you can reference a detailed timeline in an appendix to keep the letter short.

Example:

> "On April 2, 2025, I requested a referral to neurology for worsening migraines. My primary care provider placed the consult on April 5. Since then, I have made three follow-up inquiries via secure messaging and one phone call to the clinic. As of today, nearly eight weeks later, I have received no update or appointment scheduling."

3. Policy Violation: What Rule Was Broken

This is the most important section. Clearly cite the VA directive or federal statute that applies, and explain how the VA's actions failed to comply.

Example:

> "According to VHA Directive 1003.04, Paragraph 2(l)(3), Patient Advocates are required to provide prompt and thorough responses to Veteran complaints. I reported this issue to the Patient Advocate Office on May 6, but have not received any follow-up, which contradicts this policy. Additionally, VHA policy requires timely coordination with service lines to resolve access issues — this has not occurred."

4. Impact: How It Affects You

Briefly explain how the delay, denial, or mishandling has affected your health, access to care, or trust in the system. Avoid exaggeration — stick to clear, direct statements.

Example:

> *"As a result of this delay, my migraines have worsened, and I have had to seek non-VA urgent care twice. The lack of communication has also created significant stress and confusion about how to proceed with my treatment."*

5. Resolution: What You Are Requesting

Make a specific, reasonable request. If you are unsure what resolution is appropriate, ask for a review and policy-based response.

Example:

> *"I am requesting that this matter be reviewed by appropriate leadership and that I be contacted within 5 business days with a resolution. I would also like a written explanation of how this delay complies with VA scheduling policy."*

6. Closing Statement

Finish with a professional closing that emphasizes your expectation of a timely response and reiterates your intent to escalate if necessary.

Example:

> *"I appreciate your attention to this matter and hope it can be resolved quickly. If no resolution is provided, I will escalate this complaint to the facility director and, if necessary, to VISN leadership and congressional oversight."*

Checklist: Structuring Your Complaint — Step-by-Step

Use the 5-Part Complaint Structure:

1. Intro: What This Is and Why It Matters
    - ☐ Start with a clear, one-sentence summary of the problem.
    - ☐ State what you are asking for (investigation, response, correction, etc.).
2. What Happened
    - ☐ Describe the situation clearly, including who, what, when, and where.
    - ☐ Keep it factual and focused.
3. What Should Have Happened
    - ☐ Quote or paraphrase the relevant policy or directive.
    - ☐ Briefly explain how the VA's actions violated that standard.
4. What You Did to Resolve It
    - ☐ Mention previous complaints, Patient Advocate involvement, or attempts to escalate.
    - ☐ Include dates and who you spoke to (if possible).
5. What You're Asking for Now
    - ☐ Clearly state what outcome you are requesting.
    - ☐ Be reasonable and solution-focused (e.g., re-review, correction, response from leadership).

Section 4 — Writing an Effective Congressional Inquiry Request

A congressional inquiry is not just another complaint — it's a formal request for oversight from an elected official. That means your request needs to be sharp, focused, and fully documented. While the congressional office may help you draft the final submission, the more prepared and policy-backed your initial request is, the more effective it will be.

Here's how to structure your congressional inquiry request:

1. Start with a Clear Ask

Begin your message by stating exactly what you're asking your member of Congress to do — typically, to initiate a congressional inquiry with the Department of Veterans Affairs regarding a specific issue.

Example:

> "I am requesting a formal congressional inquiry into the ongoing delay in access to neurology care at the Bay Pines VA Medical Center. I believe this delay violates VA access-to-care standards and may be placing my health at risk."

2. Briefly Describe the Issue

Summarize the problem in a few sentences. Focus on the core issue, not every detail.

Example:

> "I was referred for specialty care on [date], but the appointment was never scheduled. Despite repeated follow-ups with my primary care team and the Patient Advocate's office, I have received no appointment or explanation. My symptoms have worsened in the meantime, and I have documentation from my provider stating that a timely neurology consult is medically necessary."

3. Explain What You've Already Done

Congressional offices want to see that you've tried to resolve the matter through normal VA channels first. Include who you contacted, when, and what happened (or didn't happen).

Example:

> "I contacted the Patient Advocate on [date], followed up on [date], and then escalated the issue to the facility director's office on [date]. To date, no action has been taken and I've received no explanation for the delay."

4. Reference Policy or Law

Link your complaint to a known regulation or directive, if possible. This gives the congressional staff a clear basis for their inquiry.

Example:

> "VHA Directive 1230 requires the VA to provide timely access to specialty care, and VHA Directive 1003.04 outlines the duties of Patient Advocates to coordinate resolution of complaints and access issues. Both of these obligations appear to have been disregarded in this case."

5. Attach Evidence, Organized as Appendices

Keep your main message concise and reference any supporting evidence in an attached appendix. This can include screenshots of Secure Messages, copies of referrals, provider notes, and your prior complaints.

Example:

> *"Please see Appendix A for a timeline of my contacts with the VA, and Appendix B for medical documentation showing the clinical need for timely neurology care."*

6. Include Your Full Contact Information

This includes your address, phone number, email, last four digits of your SSN, and your VA facility and PACT team information. Most congressional offices require this to verify your identity and authorize a case inquiry.

Every Veteran case is different, but strong complaints tend to follow similar structures. Appendix C gives you working templates and real examples you can adapt to your situation. They are based on what has actually worked for Veterans who pushed their concerns to VA leadership, VISN, the Office of the Inspector General (OIG), and Congressional offices.

Each example provided is structured with clarity, professionalism, and a clear connection to VA policy or federal law. Use them as a foundation — just swap in your specific facts, timelines, and policy citations as needed.

When Veterans write complaints backed by policy, clarity, and purpose, they transform frustration into leverage. A well-structured, well-documented complaint is more than a grievance — it's a formal challenge to a system that promised timely, coordinated, and respectful care. And when your complaint is grounded in the VA's own rulebook, it's no longer your word against theirs — it's a matter of compliance.

But as you've likely experienced, a strong complaint doesn't always lead to immediate resolution. Sometimes it's met with silence. Sometimes with deflection. That's when the second half of the strategy begins.

The next chapter will show you how to follow up when they don't respond, how to escalate without starting over, and how to use the very act of being ignored as evidence of deeper failure. Because in a system that often counts on Veterans giving up, your persistence is power. Your paper trail becomes pressure. And when you stay engaged — professionally, strategically, and relentlessly — you don't just hold the system accountable.

You change it.

Checklist: Congressional Inquiry Request
Use this checklist to ensure your congressional request is complete, focused, and ready for action:

- ☐ **Clear and Specific Ask:** Clearly state what you are asking the congressional office to do (e.g., initiate an inquiry)

- ☐ **Succinct Summary of the Problem:** Describe the issue in 3–4 sentences, focusing on what happened and why it matters

- ☐ **Evidence of Attempted Resolution** Explain what steps you took within the VA system and what responses (or lack thereof) you received

- ☐ **Policy or Law Cited** Include at least one reference to a VA directive or federal statute that was violated

- ☐ **Appendices Attached** Include relevant supporting documents (referrals, messages, notes) as organized appendices

- ☐ **Contact and Identification Info Included** Include your full name, address, phone, email, last four of SSN, VA facility, and PACT team

Chapter 11: Following Up and Maintaining Pressure

Writing a strong complaint is the first step toward accountability — but it's not always the last. In the VA system, complaints can be ignored, delayed, or casually dismissed unless the Veteran keeps pushing. This is where many give up — not because they were wrong, but because the system quietly waited them out.

That's why follow-up isn't optional. It's the second half of the strategy — and often the part that makes the biggest impact.

This chapter is about what happens after you've spoken up. You'll learn how to follow up with clarity, how to track timelines and responses, and how to escalate when silence becomes the only answer you get. You'll see how to use your documentation as evidence, how to hold leadership accountable by name and policy, and how to shift from requesting help to demanding answers.

VA policy isn't a suggestion. And when you cite the rules, ask the right questions, and refuse to let your complaint be buried, you become more than a patient — you become a force the system has to reckon with.

This is how you keep the pressure on — and how you protect both yourself and the next Veteran who's about to face the same barrier.

Section 1 — Follow-Up Matters: Why Persistence Wins

Writing a clear, policy-based complaint is a powerful first move — but what you do next often determines whether your case gets resolved or gets buried. The hard truth is this: many VA complaints are ignored not because they're weak, but because the system is betting you won't follow up. In too many cases, silence becomes the VA's default response strategy.

That's why your second message — and your third if needed — matters more than most Veterans realize. In a bureaucracy that moves slowly, persistence signals something important: you're not going away. And that changes everything.

Silence Is Not Resolution

The absence of a response is not a resolution. It's a tactic. Whether intentional or due to overwhelmed staff, silence from the VA becomes a form of passive resistance. But here's the key — the longer your complaint remains unanswered, the stronger your case becomes for escalation. When you follow up in writing, you're not only advancing your issue — you're creating a documented trail of neglect that can later be used as formal evidence.

Timelines Matter — And the Clock Is Ticking

While VA policies don't always give firm deadlines for complaint resolution, VHA Directive 1003.04 makes it clear that complaints must be "resolved in a timely manner." That phrase has weight. A two-week delay without communication? That's not timely. A month of silence? That's a failure of the Patient Advocacy Program.

Track your timelines. If you received no update within 10–14 business days, it's appropriate — and strategic — to send a follow-up message that:

- Reiterates your original concern
- Documents the lack of response
- Cites the obligation under policy for timely action
- Politely demands next steps or escalation

Follow-Up Creates Leverage

Every follow-up message strengthens your position. It shows you're serious, organized, and building a paper trail. Staff may be tempted to dismiss your first message. They'll think twice when they realize you're documenting every gap and delay.

And if you ever need to escalate to a Facility Director, VISN, Member of Congress, or the Office of Inspector General, your follow-ups become key exhibits. They show that you gave the system a fair chance to respond — and it failed.

> *"This is my second written request. As of today, I have not received a response to my original message sent on [Date]. This matter remains unresolved, and I request clarification under VHA Directive 1003.04 regarding the expected timeline for resolution and appropriate service recovery."*

This type of follow-up is not aggressive — it's professional. It signals that you know your rights, and that you're holding the system to its own standard.

Persistence Is Not Being Difficult — It's Being Strategic

Veterans are often told, directly or indirectly, that persistence makes them "*difficult*." That's not true — and don't let anyone convince you otherwise. Following up is exactly what the VA expects of an engaged, informed patient. You're not just protecting yourself — you're also exposing a system that counts on silence to bury problems.

The next sections will show you how to use that persistence as fuel — through strategic language, properly escalated messages, and a complaint log that becomes your greatest asset when the system continues to fall short.

Section 2 — Using Escalation Language Effectively

When a complaint is ignored or delayed, your next move needs to be more than just a repeat — it needs to escalate. Not with emotion, but with precision. The way you write your follow-up message can dramatically influence whether your issue is finally addressed or continues to be brushed aside.

This section gives you the tools to escalate your message without sounding confrontational — and shows you how to use language that commands attention and triggers accountability.

Why Escalation Language Matters

VA staff are trained to recognize certain terms that signal risk, non-compliance, or leadership involvement. These are not just buzzwords — they're built into VA directives, reporting systems, and performance metrics. When you use the VA's own language, you shift your follow-up from a "*reminder*" to a documented compliance issue.

- You are no longer *asking* for help.
- You are *reminding* them they are out of compliance.
- And you are *putting* leadership on notice — in writing.

Phrases That Trigger Action

Use these phrases in your subject lines or early in the message body to signal that this isn't just a routine inquiry anymore:

- Second Request – Unresolved Complaint Regarding [Issue]
- Escalation – Non-Compliance with VHA Directive 1003.04
- Request for Written Explanation – VA Failure to Follow Service Recovery Policy
- This issue may warrant VISN-level review due to lack of local resolution

And in the body of your message:

- "*This matter appears to require escalation under VA policy due to lack of resolution within a reasonable timeframe.*"
- "*I am requesting a written explanation under VHA Directive 1003.04 outlining why this complaint has not been resolved.*"
- "*This is now a repeat failure. I request this issue be flagged as a pattern under your Process Improvement responsibilities.*"
- "*If I don't receive a formal response within 10 business days, I will elevate this concern to VISN and my congressional office.*"

These are not threats — they are strategic notices that you understand how VA policy works and you're using it appropriately.

Make the Subject Line Work for You

When you send secure messages through MyHealtheVet or write to a Patient Advocate or clinic supervisor, your subject line matters. It's the first thing they see — and a strong subject line can move your message to the top of the queue.

Examples:

    POOR - Checking In Again

    GOOD - Second Request: Referral Delay – Neurology Consult Missing

    POOR - Follow-up on MRI

    GOOD - Policy Violation – MRI Result Not Communicated Within Required Timeframe (VHA Dir. 1003)

This is how you take control of the narrative. You're not "following up." You're applying pressure in a way that VA staff and leadership are trained to recognize.

Escalation Is a Process — Not a Threat

You're not threatening to go above someone's head — you're following the VA's own escalation structure. VHA Directive 1003.04 makes it clear that unresolved complaints are to be tracked, monitored, and escalated when appropriate. You are doing your part in that chain of accountability.

Escalation also sets you up for the next phase — reaching out to higher-level officials or oversight bodies. When you've used policy terms and escalation language at the local level, you can later show that you made every effort to resolve the matter internally before going higher. That's what gives your case credibility.

Pro Tip: Use Escalation Language in Writing, Not Over the Phone

When you use these terms in secure messages, emails, or letters, you create a documented trail that you can later forward or attach to your complaint if escalation is needed. Verbal escalation gets forgotten or denied. Written escalation is permanent.

In the next section, we'll walk through **who** to escalate to — and how to do it effectively at every level, from clinic supervisor to VISN leadership.

Section 3 — When to Involve Leadership

When frontline VA staff fail to resolve your issue, ignore your complaint, or act outside policy — and your follow-up messages are met with silence or vague assurances — it's time to escalate beyond them. This isn't being impatient. It's following the very accountability structure the VA created.

This section will show you how to identify the right points of escalation, what to include in your message, and how to make your request stand out from routine grievances.

Who Counts as Leadership?

There are four main layers of escalation within the VA health care system. Use them progressively — or jump levels when the failure is clear and serious.

1. Clinic or Service Line Supervisor
   Direct supervisor of the team that failed you (e.g., Primary Care Chief, Specialty Clinic Supervisor)

2. Facility-Level Leadership
   Includes the Patient Advocate Supervisor, Chief of Staff, or Medical Center Director

3. VISN Leadership
   The Veterans Integrated Service Network Director and Quality Management Officer who oversee multiple VA facilities in your region

4. National Oversight and External Watchdogs
   The Under Secretary for Health, VA Central Office, or oversight bodies like the Office of Inspector General (OIG) and Congressional staff

When to Escalate

Escalation is appropriate when:

- Your initial complaint has received no response within 10–14 business days

- A Patient Advocate fails to act, communicate, or explain policy

- The service line claims your issue is "resolved" without actually fixing the problem

- The same issue keeps happening, even after previous complaints

- Staff deny care, access, or form completion contrary to VA policy

- You've documented two or more failed attempts to resolve the issue

If you're unsure, use this simple rule: If you would advise another Veteran in your position to escalate — then escalate.

How to Escalate Professionally

Escalation doesn't mean sounding angry. It means being clear, specific, and grounded in policy. Below is a sample email to a Facility Director of Service Chief:

> Subject: Escalation – Unresolved Access to Neurology Care (VHA Dir. 1003.04, 1003)
>
> Dear [Director's Name],
>
> I am writing to formally escalate a patient care issue that remains unresolved despite multiple prior attempts. I submitted a secure message on [date], followed by a Patient Advocate complaint on [date], regarding a referral delay for neurology care.
>
> As of today, I have not received any update, action, or explanation. This matter appears to violate the timeliness and service recovery provisions outlined in VHA Directives 1003 and 1003.04.
>
> I request immediate attention to this matter and a written response outlining what steps will be taken to resolve it. If unresolved within 10 business days, I intend to elevate this complaint to VISN leadership and my congressional representative.
>
> Respectfully,
> [Your Name]
> [Last Four of SSN or DOB]
> [VA Medical Center Name]

How to Find Contact Information

- **Facility Director Emails** are often listed on each VA medical center's webpage

- **VISN Director and staff contacts** can be found at: https://department.va.gov/integrated-service-networks/

- If unavailable, call the VA's main facility line and ask for the **Office of the Director** or **Patient Advocate Supervisor**

Don't Ask — Assert

Instead of:

"Would you be willing to look into this?"

Use:

"This issue requires executive leadership review under VHA Directive 1003.04, which places accountability for unresolved complaints directly with facility leadership."

You are not requesting a favor. You are invoking an obligation.

In the next section, you'll learn how to create a **Complaint Log** — a powerful tool for strengthening your credibility and providing leadership with a clear, undeniable paper trail.

Section 4 — Creating and Maintaining a Complaint Log

A well-kept complaint log is the advocacy equivalent of a flight recorder: it captures who said what, when they said it, and how (or whether) they followed through. When leadership finally reviews your case—or when an oversight body asks for "all correspondence"—this log turns vague memories into hard facts.

Why a Log Changes the Power Dynamic

Without a Log	With a Log
"I called a few times and no one got back to me."	"On **April 8** at **14:15**, I phoned Neurology; **Ms. Flores** stated the consult 'was still pending,' contradicting CPRS notes printed the same day."
Staff deny delays or blame other departments.	You cite exact dates, names, and relevant policy each step of the way.
Leadership can minimize the issue as an isolated case.	Your timeline reveals a pattern— evidence of systemic failure, not a one-off glitch.

What to Track (The 4-Point Method)

1. **Date & Time** – When the interaction happened.
2. **Action/Contact** – Call, secure message, walk-in, mailed letter, etc.
3. **VA Response (or Lack Thereof)** – Who responded, what they said, or note *"No response"* after 10 business days.
4. **Policy Reference** – The directive, CFR, or statute you cited—or that they ignored.

Pro Tip: Attach or link supporting documents (screenshots, after-visit summaries, letters). Label them "Exhibit A," "Exhibit B," etc., so you can quickly drop them into an escalation email.

Template You Can Start Using Today (see Appendix E for more details)

Date	Action Taken	VA Response	Policy Involved	Next Step
07 Apr 25	Secure msg to PCP re: lost neurology consult	No response by 17 Apr 25	VHA Dir 1003 (Timeliness)	Follow-up msg, CC Patient Advocate
18 Apr 25 09:20	Call to Patient Advocate Office – spoke w/ Mr. James	Stated "consults are backlog-related" but offered no ETA	38 U.S.C. § 7309A, VHA Dir 1003.04	Email summary to Mr. James; request written plan
30 Apr 25	Email to Service Chief (Neuro) labelled **Escalation**	Awaiting reply	VHA Dir 1232(2) (Referral processing)	Escalate to Med Ctr Director if no reply by 10 May

Digital vs. Paper

- **Digital spreadsheet** (Excel, Google Sheets) makes sorting and filtering easy, and you can attach files or cloud links.
- **Notebook** works if you're more comfortable handwriting; just photograph or scan pages so you can email them later.
- **MyHealtheVet Download**: You can download your secure-message history to attach as exhibits—another built-in audit trail.

How Often to Update

- **Immediately** after any call or clinic visit—while details are fresh.
- **Weekly** review: highlight entries older than 14 days with no response; these become your next follow-ups.
- **Before every escalation**: skim the log, copy the most relevant line items into your email so leadership sees the time stamps.

Turning the Log Into Leverage

When you escalate, paste a concise excerpt:

> *"Attached timeline shows four unanswered contacts between 07 Apr 25 and 30 Apr 25. This pattern violates the timeliness requirements in VHA Directive 1003. I request immediate service-recovery action and a written plan of correction."*

Leadership now confronts hard data, not anecdote. Ignoring that data risks their own performance metrics—and they know it.

With your complaint log in place, you're ready for the next level: using the VA's silence (or inadequate replies) as evidence to press VISN leadership, Congress, or the Office of Inspector General.

Section 5 — Using Silence as Leverage

At the VA, silence is rarely accidental. Whether it's a missed message, an unanswered call, or a Patient Advocate who stops responding, that silence becomes a tactic — one that delays resolution and wears Veterans down.

But silence isn't just frustrating. It's evidence. And when you know how to use it, it becomes one of your strongest tools in escalating your case and triggering oversight.

Silence Is a Compliance Failure — Not a Dead End

VA policy doesn't permit "ghosting." VHA Directive 1003 and 1003.04 both require:

- Timely resolution of complaints
- Clear, ongoing communication
- Documentation of follow-up steps

When the VA fails to respond within a reasonable timeframe (generally 10–14 business days), that's not just poor service — it's a violation of their own patient experience obligations.

> *"No response to a formal complaint submitted in writing is a failure of process, not a scheduling backlog."*

Reframing the Silence in Your Follow-Up

Don't beg for answers. Instead, reframe the silence as a failure of the system — and flag it as such.

Example Language:

> *"As of [today's date], I have received no response to my written complaint submitted on [original date], despite follow-ups on [date1, date2]."*

This lack of response appears to violate VA's obligation under VHA Directive 1003.04 to resolve complaints in a timely and documented manner. I am now escalating this issue for leadership review and service recovery."

Attach the Timeline — Then Let Silence Speak for You

Include a few key lines from your complaint log showing exactly how long you've waited and how many times you've followed up.

Example:

Date	Action	Response
Apr 7	Secure message to PCP	No response (10+ business days)
Apr 18	Call to Patient Advocate	Stated they would follow up — no further contact
Apr 30	Written escalation to Service Chief	No reply by May 10

Then write:

"Given the above, this now constitutes a documented pattern of inaction. I am requesting formal service recovery and, if unresolved within 10 days, I will elevate this matter to VISN 08 and the Office of the Inspector General."

This takes the burden off you — and puts it squarely on the system that failed to respond.

Use Silence to Justify Escalation

When you go to a VISN Director, a Congressman, or OIG, you'll be expected to show you tried to resolve the issue internally first. Silence becomes your justification:

- *"I attempted resolution through proper channels but received no reply."*

- *"I submitted [X] messages and received either no response or vague non-answers."*

- *"There is no documented resolution, despite multiple formal attempts."*

The more silent they are, the louder your case becomes when you bring it to higher levels.

Pro Tip: Silence Doesn't Expire — **It Accumulates**

> Even if a VA employee responds *later*, the delay itself is still part of the record. Late action doesn't erase the fact that the system failed to respond when it should have.
>
> So don't delete those complaint log entries or change *"No Response"* to *"Resolved."* Add a new line — and keep building your case.

In the final section of this chapter, we'll explore how to recognize when it's time to take your complaint beyond the facility altogether — and exactly how to do it.

Section 6 — What If Nothing Works? Next Steps

Sometimes, despite your best efforts — despite writing a clear complaint, citing policy, tracking timelines, following up, and escalating — the system still doesn't respond. Or worse, it responds with excuses, misdirection, or empty reassurances. When that happens, it's not the end. It's the beginning of the next phase: external pressure and formal oversight.

This section walks you through where to go when the VA at the facility level has failed — and how to escalate strategically, not just reactively.

You Gave the System a Chance — Now Use That to Your Advantage

Everything you've documented so far proves one thing: you gave the VA every opportunity to fix the problem. You followed the chain of command. You used their rules. You acted in good faith. That history gives you the credibility — and the justification — to take your case beyond the walls of the VA.

Now it's time to act like it.

Where to Go When the Facility Stops Responding

1. VISN Director

    - Every VA facility belongs to a regional **Veterans Integrated Service Network** (VISN).
    - VISN Directors oversee all operations and patient experience failures within their region.
    - You can escalate unresolved complaints directly to them with documentation of delays and policy violations.
    - Find your VISN and leadership team here: https://department.va.gov/integrated-service-networks/

2. Your Member of Congress

    - Every VA Medical Center has a Congressional Liaison Office.

    - When a Congressman's office submits an inquiry on your behalf, the VA is obligated to respond — usually within 10–14 business days.

    - Include a cover letter with:

        o A concise timeline of events

        o Copies of unanswered complaints or policy violations

        o The specific outcome you're requesting (e.g., specialty care approval, medical record amendment, accountability action)

3. Office of Inspector General (OIG)

    - The VA OIG investigates waste, fraud, abuse, and serious breakdowns in care or accountability.

    - If your issue involves:

        o Systematic neglect

        o Falsified records

        o Patterned mismanagement

        o Unaddressed failures after escalation
        ...then the OIG may initiate a formal review.

    - Online complaint portal: https://www.va.gov/oig/hotline/default.asp

4. VA Central Office – Under Secretary for Health

    - You can send documentation of unresolved failures to the national leadership office of the VHA.

    - Keep it brief, professional, and evidence-backed.

    - They rarely respond personally but may initiate internal audits or refer your complaint back down with "visibility," which forces faster action.

Chapter 11

How to Present a High-Level Complaint

When escalating externally:

- **Lead with the failure**: "*Despite five attempts over 45 days to resolve this issue internally, no corrective action has been taken.*"
- Include your complaint **log** or a summary **timeline**
- **Cite policy** directly: "*This violates VHA Directive 1003.04 regarding timely resolution and escalation obligations.*"
- **Make your request specific**: Don't just say "*please help.*" Say, "*I am requesting a formal review of this breakdown and corrective action by leadership.*"

Protect Yourself — But Also Protect Others

When the VA fails one Veteran, it often fails many. Your complaint — when elevated correctly — becomes more than personal advocacy. It becomes evidence of systemic failure. And if handled properly, it can trigger audits, training changes, leadership reviews, or even national policy updates.

That's why your documentation, your tone, and your persistence matter. You're not just fighting for yourself. You're lighting a path for the Veteran who comes next.

Persistence doesn't make you a troublemaker — it makes you an advocate. Silence from the VA doesn't mean you're wrong. It means you're being ignored — and now, you have the tools to change that.

You've built a complete framework for holding the VA accountable at the local and regional levels. You know how to write effective complaints, follow up when they're ignored, escalate when the system stalls, and present a strong, documented case to leadership and external watchdogs.

But your most powerful tool is knowledge — not just of what went wrong, but of what was supposed to happen.
That's what the next chapters deliver. These aren't about storytelling or tactics. They're about mastering the rules of engagement — the actual laws and policies that govern your care, define your rights, and bind VA staff to their duties.

Because when you know the policies better than the people who are paid to follow them, you don't just complain — you win.

PART IV

Taking Control of the Record

"What the VA writes about you can help you — or it can quietly ruin everything. And unless you check, you may never know the difference."

If VA staff get the record wrong, your care, benefits, and credibility all suffer. And they often do it without asking a single question.

This section is about reclaiming your medical record as your voice — and not letting others define your condition, your story, or your capabilities through false or careless entries. From form completion refusals to dangerous intake notes, you'll learn what can go wrong in VA documentation, why it matters so deeply, and what rights you have to correct it.

You'll discover:

- How to compel your providers to complete forms under VHA Directive 1134

- How to challenge false documentation through formal amendment requests

- What to look for in your record — with real-world examples of hidden harm

- Why routine entries like "no ADL changes" or "functioning effectively" can quietly undermine your entire case for care and support

This part of the book is personal — because many of these failures are buried in plain sight, repeated visit after visit, and left unchallenged. But now that you know what to look for, you won't make the same mistake.

Your record is your evidence. And you deserve to make sure it reflects the truth.

Chapter 12: Requesting Medical Statements and Form Completion

For many Veterans, a completed medical form can determine access to life-changing benefits — from disability compensation and Social Security to family leave and housing support. Yet too often, VA providers refuse to complete these forms or claim they are not allowed to. That is not just incorrect — it violates VA policy and your legal right to care.

VHA Directive 1134(2) establishes that VA providers are required to complete medical forms and statements that are necessary for Veterans to obtain services, benefits, or protections. This policy is not optional — it is part of your official VA **medical benefits package**, as defined by **38 C.F.R. § 17.38(a)(1)(xv)**. This regulation makes it clear: the completion of medical forms is a covered benefit when based on a provider's examination or knowledge of your condition.

Whether it's a **Disability Benefits Questionnaire (DBQ)**, a **Family Medical Leave Act form**, or an **Aid & Attendance certification**, your treating provider has a duty to help. They must either complete the form, refer it appropriately, or provide a written reason why they cannot.

This chapter walks you through exactly what VHA Directive 1134(2) requires, how to assert your rights when providers push back, and what steps to take if the VA fails to comply. With the law and policy on your side, you're not asking for a favor — you're demanding what's already yours.

Section 1 — DBQs and Form Completion by VA Providers

Veterans frequently need documentation from their VA providers to access critical services — disability benefits, leave from work, housing accommodations, or legal protections. For years, inconsistent practices and misinformation led many providers to deny these requests or refer Veterans elsewhere. VHA **Directive 1134(2)** changed that — and it's not new.

This directive has been in effect since **August 2016**. That means VA providers and leadership have had nearly a decade to implement its guidance. Yet, many Veterans still hear the same line: *"We don't do that here."* This response isn't just wrong — it reflects a failure of leadership, training, and accountability. The VA has had ample time to train its staff, but the burden continues to fall on Veterans to cite the rules and push for enforcement.

VHA Directive 1134(2) requires VA clinicians to complete medical statements and forms that relate to a Veteran's current health condition — including documents requested by **other federal agencies, state programs, private insurers, attorneys, or employers**. This is not limited to VA-related benefits. It applies broadly.

Most importantly, the right to have these forms completed is backed by regulation — specifically **38 C.F.R. § 17.38(a)(1)(xv)**. This regulation defines the scope of the VA's medical benefits package, and it explicitly includes:

> "Completion of forms (e.g., family medical leave, life insurance, and private disability insurance forms) based on an examination or knowledge of the Veteran's condition."

In other words, when a VA provider has direct knowledge of your condition — either from treating you or reviewing your medical record — they are **required** to complete forms related to your care. It is not a discretionary service. It is a benefit you are entitled to receive under federal regulation.

VHA Directive 1134(2) reinforces this legal foundation by:

- Requiring every VA facility to assign a Medical Statements and Forms Point of Contact (MS&F POC)
- Establishing a **20-business-day** turnaround standard for form completion
- Mandating a **reconsideration process** if a provider initially refuses
- Clarifying that providers must complete **any form related to the Veteran's medical condition**, regardless of the requesting agency

Understanding this policy — and the regulation behind it — gives you the leverage you need to hold the VA accountable when a provider says "*we can't do that here.*" Yes, they can. And under federal law, they must. And when a provider acts surprised when presented the directive, remember: this policy is not new. They should know better. And now — so do you.

Section 2 — What VA Providers Are Required to Do

VHA Directive 1134(2) is unambiguous: when a Veteran requests the completion of a medical statement or form related to their care, the VA provider is expected to comply — not ignore, delay, or deflect. The directive sets a clear expectation that form completion is **part of clinical care**, and providers must act in good faith to assist.

What Must Be Completed

VA providers are required to complete medical statements and forms that meet the following criteria:

- The form relates to a medical condition for which the provider has direct knowledge or is currently treating the Veteran.

- The form is necessary for the Veteran to access benefits, accommodations, or legal protections — whether VA-sponsored or external.

- The form requires a clinical judgment, not a legal or administrative decision.

This includes, but is not limited to:

- VA Disability Benefits Questionnaires (DBQs)
- Social Security Disability forms
- Aid and Attendance or Housebound benefit evaluations
- Family and Medical Leave Act (FMLA) forms
- State disability applications
- Employer accommodation forms
- Attorney-generated functional assessments

If a provider has direct clinical knowledge of your condition, they are obligated to complete these forms **to the best of their ability**.

The Provider's Obligation

According to VHA Directive 1134(2), providers must:

1. Review and complete the form based on medical knowledge of the Veteran's condition (1134(2) Sec 4).

2. **Respond within 20 business days** from the date the completed form is received by the VA (not from the date the Veteran made the request) (1134(2) Sec 5(d)(2)).

3. **Forward the form** to the facility's **Medical Statements and Forms Point of Contact (MS&F POC)** if the provider cannot complete it themselves (1134(2) Sec 5(e)(3)).

4. **Provide written notice** if the form cannot be completed — including the reason and what alternate options exist (1134(2) Sec 5(d)(1)(d)(4)).

Providers are not allowed to ignore the request or refer it externally without attempting to resolve it through the MS&F POC or by seeking reconsideration.

Not Discretionary — It's Policy

Some providers still claim:

"*We don't do those here,*" or "*We're not allowed to fill that out.*"

VHA Directive 1134(2) makes it clear: **those statements are false.** The completion of valid medical forms is a covered clinical service under **38 C.F.R. § 17.38(a)(1)(xv)**. It is part of the medical benefits package that every Veteran enrolled in VA health care is entitled to receive. It is no different than getting lab work, medication, or imaging — if it relates to your condition and helps secure care or benefits, it must be addressed.

In the next section, we'll look at the exact role of the Medical Statements and Forms Point of Contact — and how they are supposed to help resolve delays and provider refusals.

Section 3 — The Medical Statements and Forms Point of Contact (MS&F POC)

VHA Directive 1134(2) requires that every VA medical center and larger community-based outpatient clinic (CBOC) designate a Medical Statements and Forms Point of Contact (MS&F POC). This role is not optional. It is mandated by national VA policy and plays a critical part in ensuring Veterans receive the documentation they need without unnecessary delay or confusion.

Who Is the MS&F POC?

The MS&F POC is the facility's **subject matter expert** on VHA Directive 1134(2). Their job is to:

- Serve as a central coordinator for all form and medical statement requests
- Assist providers in completing forms when needed
- Facilitate alternate solutions if the original provider cannot complete the form
- Ensure timely responses in accordance with the 20-business-day standard
- Educate VA staff about their obligations under this directive

This person is often housed within the Release of Information (ROI) department, Patient Administration, or Medical Administration. However, some facilities may assign the duty elsewhere — what matters is that the role exists and is functional.

How to Find Your MS&F POC

Unfortunately, VA facilities do not publish directories listing MS&F POCs, and many front-line staff aren't even aware the position exists — which itself is a policy compliance failure. Here's how to find yours:

1. Start with the ROI office: Ask if they can direct you to the MS&F POC.
2. Try Patient Advocacy: If ROI is unhelpful, ask the Patient Advocate to identify the MS&F POC.
3. Escalate to the Chief of Health Administration Services (HAS): If no one seems to know, ask to speak with HAS leadership.

They are responsible for administrative compliance with VHA directives.

4. Request in writing: If needed, file a written request under VHA Directive 1605.01 to obtain the name and contact of the designated MS&F POC under your patient rights to information access.

If your facility truly has not assigned one — or refuses to tell you who it is — you can raise that as a policy violation complaint using Chapter 9 strategies.

What the MS&F POC Can Do (and What They Can't)

What they can do:

- Help locate the correct provider to complete the form
- Coordinate referrals if the original provider is unavailable or unwilling
- Ensure the form is routed through proper channels and timelines are met
- Advise Veterans and staff about VHA Directive 1134(2) and CFR 17.38

What they can't do:

- Complete forms themselves (unless they are a licensed provider)
- Make determinations outside their clinical or administrative scope
- Override medical judgment — but they *can* escalate refusals for reconsideration

The MS&F POC is not a loophole — they are a solution built into VA policy to make sure Veterans are not abandoned when their provider won't cooperate or when bureaucratic confusion gets in the way.

Section 4 — What to Do When a VA Provider Refuses

Even though VHA Directive 1134(2) has been in place since 2016, many providers still seem unaware of its existence—or pretend it doesn't apply to them. That's not your problem. The directive is national policy, and it *does* apply. And if your provider refuses to complete a legitimate form or medical statement, the VA has specific procedures that must be followed.

Here's what to do:

1. Confirm the Request Meets VHA Directive 1134(2)

Your request must involve one of the following:

- A VA form (like Aid and Attendance, DBQs, Clothing Allowance, etc.)
- A non-VA form that relates to your health condition or functional status (e.g., FMLA, SSA disability, state benefit forms, etc.)
- A medical statement related to your current medical condition, diagnosis, prognosis, or ability to function

If your request meets these criteria, then VHA Directive 1134(2) **requires** providers to help, unless doing so would:

- Fall outside their clinical expertise
- Require specialized certification not available at the facility
- Create a conflict of interest (such as concealed carry permit forms)
- Disrupt the therapeutic relationship (more common in mental health)

If your request doesn't meet the criteria, ask your provider to explain why it falls outside the directive—and ask for that explanation in writing.

2. Ask for Reconsideration

If your provider refuses, ask for the matter to be **formally reconsidered**. VHA Directive 1134(2) is explicit:

> "*The facility must ensure there is a process in place for reconsideration when a provider refuses to issue a medical statement or complete a VA or non-VA form on behalf of a Veteran or if a Veteran objects to the content of a completed form.*" (1134(2) (5)(d)(3))

Ask your provider who is responsible for that process at your facility. If they don't know, escalate to the Patient Advocate's Office or the Release of Information (ROI) Office.

3. Contact the Medical Statements and Forms Point of Contact (MS&F POC)

Every VA medical center and larger CBOC is required to have a **Medical Statements and Forms Point of Contact (MS&F POC)**. This individual is trained on this directive and can:

- Clarify which forms fall under provider obligations
- Help resolve provider refusals
- Guide you to alternative options if needed

You can ask ROI or Patient Advocacy for the contact info for your facility's MS&F POC.

4. Escalate If Necessary

If your provider refuses without proper justification—or if you're ignored—follow your complaint strategy (see Chapter 4). In your complaint, quote the directive directly:

> "*Except when specifically prohibited, it is VHA policy that providers, when requested, must assist patients in completion of VA and non-VA medical forms and provide medical statements with respect to the patient's medical condition and functionality.*"
> — VHA Directive 1134(2), Section 4

And if the denial is based on something like "We don't do those forms," respond with:

> "This policy has been in effect since 2016. The VA is required to have staff trained and procedures in place to comply with it. A blanket refusal is not compliant."

If needed, file a formal complaint with the **VHA Office of the Medical Inspector** or contact your **Congressional Representative**. Direct them to this directive and CFR 17.38(a)(1)(xv), which includes form completion as part of the VA medical benefits package.

Section 5 — What to Do When a Provider Refuses

VHA Directive 1134(2) sets clear expectations for timeliness and communication when a Veteran submits a form or request for a medical statement. These timelines are not optional — they are binding requirements under VA policy.

The 20-Business-Day Rule

VHA Directive 1134(2) Section 5(d)(2) states:

> "The requested form or medical statement must be completed and returned to the Veteran within **20 business days** from the date it is received by the VA facility."

This means:

- The clock starts the moment VA staff receive the form, not when it's reviewed or handed to the provider.
- If a form is submitted through MyHealtheVet Secure Messaging, in person, or by mail (with tracking), you can document the submission date — and you should.
- You do not need to remind or follow up during those 20 business days unless there's no acknowledgment.

What If They Need More Time?

The directive allows flexibility when:

- A provider is on extended leave
- The form requires a consult with another specialty
- A referral is made to another provider for form completion

But delays must be documented, and you must be notified. Silence is not compliant. According to the directive, the facility must have a process in place to manage these delays and ensure the request isn't lost in the system.

You Should Expect:

- **Acknowledgment** of your request (ideally within a few days)
- **Timely form completion** within 20 business days
- **Communication** if the provider cannot complete the form
- **Reconsideration** if your request is denied

If any of those steps are missing, you have a policy violation — and you can escalate.

How to Document and Track the Timeline

To hold the VA accountable, keep the following:

- A dated copy of your completed form or request
- Screenshots or printouts of secure messages or submission receipts
- A calendar reminder for the 20-business-day deadline
- Notes from any phone calls or in-person conversations

Tracking this is not about being aggressive. It's about being accurate and defensible when a follow-up or complaint is needed. Refer to the complaint log template in Appendix E for how to document noncompliance.

What If the Form Is Time-Sensitive?

Many forms — like those for FMLA, state disability, or appeal deadlines — are extremely time-sensitive. Make that clear in your submission. Include a note like:

> "*Please note this form must be returned to [agency] no later than [date]. I respectfully request priority handling in accordance with VHA Directive 1134(2).*"

The VA is not obligated to rush forms for convenience, but they are expected to accommodate time-sensitive needs when possible and clinically appropriate.

Section 6 — When to Escalate and How?

Even with a clear policy in place, Veterans are still too often met with delay, denial, or confusion when they request a medical statement or form completion. VHA Directive 1134(2) was designed to prevent that — and when the system fails to follow it, you have every right to escalate.

Escalate When:

- Your provider refuses to complete a form without a valid reason
- You receive no response within 20 business days of submission
- You are told "we don't do that here" or are referred outside the VA
- The facility has no identifiable MS&F Point of Contact (a required role)
- You are denied without being offered the reconsideration process required by the directive

These are not just bad experiences. They are violations of national VA policy and can be documented as such.

What to Say in Your Complaint

When escalating, cite both the directive and the regulation that supports it. For example:

> "I am submitting this complaint based on VHA Directive 1134(2), which requires providers to complete forms and medical statements relating to a Veteran's condition, and 38 C.F.R. § 17.38(a)(1)(xv), which includes this as part of the VA medical benefits package. The refusal to complete [form name] and the failure to provide a reconsideration process violate this policy."

Be specific, professional, and document all prior attempts to resolve the issue.

Where to Escalate

Here are your options, in the recommended order of escalation:

1. **Patient Advocate** at your VA facility
   Provide copies of your request, the missed deadline, and any refusals

2. **Release of Information (ROI) Office** or Health Administration Services (HAS)
   Ask them to confirm who the MS&F POC is and explain the delay

3. **VISN Patient Advocate or Leadership**
   If local escalation fails, raise the issue to the regional level

4. **Congressional Representative**
   Send a written summary with documentation attached and cite VHA Directive 1134(2) and 38 C.F.R. § 17.38

5. **VHA Office of the Medical Inspector or OIG (for persistent noncompliance)**
   If a pattern of disregard for this directive exists, this becomes a systemic failure

Chapter 9 of this book outlines exactly how to build an escalation package with professionalism, policy citations, and documentation.

You Shouldn't Have to Escalate — But You Can

The VA's own rules are on your side. You don't need to yell. You don't need to beg. You need to quote the policy, log the delay, and file a professional but firm complaint when they break the rules.

Every time you do, you increase the pressure on the system to change — and you make it harder for staff to ignore their obligations the next time a Veteran asks.

Know the Policy, Demand the Standard

VHA Directive 1134(2) is not a suggestion — it is binding policy that empowers you to get the documentation you need for benefits, protections, and access to care. Since 2016, every VA provider has been expected to comply with this directive. Every VA medical center has been required to designate a point of contact. And every Veteran has had the right to have their health information documented on forms that affect their lives.

Yet here we are — still having to explain the rules to the very people who are paid to follow them.

This chapter has shown you that you're not asking for a favor. You are requesting a service that is legally part of the VA's medical benefits package under 38 C.F.R. § 17.38(a)(1)(xv). The policy is on your side. The law is on your side. And now, so is your preparation.

When your provider says no, you now know what to ask, what to cite, who to contact, and how to escalate. You have the full policy. You have the right vocabulary. You are no longer defenseless.

Because when a system counts on Veterans not knowing the rules — learning the rules becomes your greatest form of leverage.

Chapter 13: Amending False or Misleading VA Medical Records

The Law Is on Your Side — Use It

Every Veteran deserves to have a medical record that is accurate, complete, and free of misleading statements. But when VA providers insert language that distorts what happened — or omit key facts — those records can cause long-term harm to your care, your reputation, and your benefits.

The good news? You have enforceable legal rights to challenge and correct those records. These rights aren't optional. They are guaranteed by **federal law** under the **Privacy Act of 1974 (5 USC § 552a)**, and they are reinforced in binding VA policy through:

- **38 CFR § 1.579** – governing how the VA must respond to correction requests

- **VA Handbook 6300.4** – detailing step-by-step amendment procedures

- **VHA Directive 1605.01** – applying those protections specifically to your VA health records

These policies grant you the right to:

- Request correction of any VA medical record you believe is inaccurate, incomplete, irrelevant, or misleading

- Receive a written response within specific timeframes (10-day acknowledgment; 30-day resolution)

- Submit a formal **Statement of Disagreement** if the VA refuses to correct the record

- Have your disagreement **permanently attached** to the contested record

- Pursue further appeal or **judicial review** if the system fails to comply

The VA cannot deny your request simply because they "*stand by the note*" or claim "*we don't change provider documentation.*" That's not how the law works — and that's not what VA policy allows.

This chapter will show you how to:

- Submit a correction request the right way
- Respond to VA delays or denials
- Challenge false or misleading entries effectively
- Use your rights to escalate and protect your record

If your VA record doesn't tell the truth, this chapter will help you demand it does — and force the system to respond when it doesn't.

Section 1 — Your Right to Request Record Corrections Under the Privacy Act and VA Policy

Most Veterans don't know that when the VA puts something false, misleading, or incomplete in their medical record, they don't have to just live with it. Federal law — specifically the **Privacy Act of 1974 (5 USC § 552a)** — gives you the legal right to request a correction. That right applies directly to VA medical records and is fully supported by VA's own rules:

- 38 CFR § 1.579
- VA Handbook 6300.4
- VHA Directive 1605.01

Together, these policies form a powerful but underused legal shield for Veterans seeking to set the record straight.

What the Law Guarantees You

Under **5 USC § 552a(d)(2)**, any individual may request the amendment of a federal record pertaining to them that they believe is:

- Inaccurate
- Irrelevant
- Untimely
- Incomplete

Chapter 13

VA medical records fall under this law because they are part of a federal system of records. That means you can legally challenge any entry that distorts the truth — even if it's just poorly worded or paints the wrong picture.

The VA is then required to:

1. Acknowledge your request within 10 business days

2. Complete a review and provide a written response within 30 business days

3. If denied, inform you of your right to submit a written Statement of Disagreement

4. Include your disagreement in any future disclosures of the disputed record

VA Policy Is Not Optional — It's Legally Binding

Each of the following VA documents enforces these rights internally:

- **38 CFR § 1.579** — Establishes the legal procedures VA must follow for amending records, including forwarding the request to the responsible official, timeframes for reply, and the right to appeal.

- **VA Handbook 6300.4** — Provides the detailed internal process for VA employees. It confirms that all requests for correction **must be reviewed by the originating office** and that the Privacy Officer is responsible for coordinating and tracking the outcome.

- **VHA Directive 1605.01** — Applies these rules specifically to health records maintained by VHA, including CPRS notes, consults, and other documentation. It emphasizes that Veterans must be informed in writing of any denial and provided instructions for submitting a disagreement.

Key Point: Nowhere in any of these policies does it say that providers are free to "*decline all changes*" or that the record "*cannot be amended.*" Those are common staff myths — and they're directly contradicted by law.

Chapter 13

You Have the Final Word in the Record

Even if the VA denies your amendment request, you are legally entitled to submit a Statement of Disagreement *5 USC § 552a(d)(3)*. This statement:

- Becomes a permanent part of your VA record
- Must be included in every future disclosure of the disputed note
- Cannot be altered or ignored by VA staff

This means you're never powerless. The VA might control what gets written — but you control what gets challenged, clarified, and recorded alongside it.

In the next section, we'll walk through **how to submit a correction request properly** — including where to send it, what to include, and how to avoid common mistakes that lead to delays or denials.

Section 2 — How to Request a Correction

The VA provides a standardized form titled **"Patient Amendment Request"** to help Veterans formally request corrections to their VA health records. This form streamlines the process and ensures that your request is handled according to the rules established in:

- **5 U.S.C. § 552a(d)** (Privacy Act of 1974)
- **38 C.F.R. § 1.579** (Amendment of Records)
- **VA Handbook 6300.4** (Processing of Privacy Act Requests)
- **VHA Directive 1605.01** (Privacy and Release of Information)

This section walks you through each part of the form, what to include, and how to submit it.

Overview: What This Form Does

The Patient Amendment Request Form allows you to:

- Identify exactly what information in your VA record you believe is **inaccurate, incomplete, or misleading**
- Specify **which VA facility** or provider created the record
- Submit **supporting documentation** to justify your request
- Ensure your request is processed by the facility's **Privacy Officer**, as required by law

How to Complete the Form — Section by Section

Top of the Form – Patient Information

Provide your identifying details, including:

- Full name
- Last 4 digits of SSN
- Date of birth
- Address, phone, and email

This information helps ensure your request is matched correctly to your record.

Question 1 – Description of the Record to Be Amended

Be specific about:

- **Which record you want amended** (e.g., "Primary Care note from Dr. Smith states ...")
- **Where it is located** (e.g., "Bay Pines VA Medical Center, under Notes")

Question 2 – Date and Time of the Entry to Be Amended

While the form only asks for the date, **including the time** helps the Privacy Officer locate the record quickly — especially if there are multiple entries on the same day.

Question 3 – Reason for the Amendment Request

Select one or more of the form's suggested reasons:

- The information is inaccurate
- The information is incomplete
- The information is irrelevant
- The information is untimely

Question 4 – How to Correct the Record

State how you want the record to be amended. Be precise. If you already quoted the original statement in Question 1, you do not need to repeat it here. Examples:

- "*Please **delete** the entire statement.*"
- "*Please **change** the statement to:* '[insert corrected language].'"
- "*Please **add** after the statement* "[missing information"]."

Note: You do not need to explain why the change is necessary here — that explanation should be included in your attached personal statement.

Question 5 – Anyone who may have received or relied on the incorrect information

This is a simple Yes/No question.

- If **No**, you may move on.
- If **Yes**, provide a list of anyone — inside or outside the VA — who may have received or acted on the incorrect information. If you need more space, attach an additional page.

Bottom of the Form

If you are the Veteran, sign and date the form.

If someone is completing the form on your behalf, they must also include:

- Printed Name of Personal Representative
- Representative's Phone Number and mailing address
- Attached proof of legal authority (such as power of attorney, legal guardianship, or official caregiver designation)

Veteran Name: _____ Date: _____

Last 4 SSN: _____ Phone Number: (____) _____

Address: _____
_____
_____

1. Description of the information/statement you are requesting to be amended (e.g., health record, lab results): *Attach a copy of record being disputed, if possible.
_____
_____
_____
_____

2. Date of the information to be amended (*This may be the date of clinic visit, date of the note, procedure or other service): _____

3. What is the reason for requesting this amendment (*Is the information inaccurate, incomplete, irrelevant, or untimely): _____

4. How should the records be stated, *please specify in writing below
   Example 1: Please change statement XYZ to the statement ABC
   Example 2: Please delete the entire statement from my health record
_____
_____
_____
_____
_____

5. Do you know of anyone who may have received or relied on the information in question? ☐ Yes ☐ No   If yes, who? _____

_____
Signature of Veteran or Personal Representative
* If you are the personal representative, please print your name, address & phone number and attach a copy of relevant legal documenqation (e.g., guardianship, POA, etc.)

Chapter 13

Attach a Copy of the Record to be Amended

Include a printed, downloaded, or screenshot copy of the VA medical record entry you want changed. The entry should clearly display:

- The **date and time** of the entry
- The name of the provider who entered it

To avoid confusion, **highlight** the part of the entry you are asking to be amended.

Attach a Personal Statement of Explanation

This is your opportunity to explain **why** the entry is wrong or misleading. Keep it factual and concise. You don't need to cite policy — just clearly explain the error and what the correct record should reflect. Examples:

- *"The note states I refused treatment, but I requested referral to a specialist."*
- *"The problem list does not reflect the diagnosis discussed with me by the provider on [date]."*
- *"The nurse intake note says I exercise three times per week, but I did not say that and I am physically unable to exercise due to my condition."*

Attach Supporting Documentation

Check the appropriate box on the form and include any documents that support your request:

- After Visit Summaries
- Secure Messages
- Past consults or referrals
- Diagnostic test results
- Personal notes or signed witness statements

These attachments increase the strength and credibility of your request.

How to Submit the Form

Send your completed amendment request to the **Privacy Officer** at the VA facility that maintains the record. You can submit it in one of the following ways:

- VA Secure Messenger (recommended)
- **In person** (ask for a date-stamped copy)
- **By mail** (use certified tracking or return receipt)

Every VA Medical Center is required to have a designated Privacy Officer. If you're unsure where to send your form, call the facility's main line or ask the Patient Advocate.

Timelines and What to Expect

VA policy requires the following:

- A written acknowledgment within 10 business days
- A written **decision within 30 business days** (with one allowable 30-day extension)
- If your request is **denied**, the VA must:
  - Provide a written explanation for the denial
  - Explain your right to submit a **Statement of Disagreement**
  - Notify you of your right to appeal to the Office of General Counsel

Keep a Copy of Everything

Make and keep a copy of:

- Your completed amendment request form
- All attachments
- Proof of submission (e.g., mail receipts, screenshots, or stamped copies)

Log all communications and follow-up in your **complaint record**, as described in Appendix E.

In the next section, we'll look at what to do when the problem isn't just an error — but a misleading or damaging entry that affects your credibility, care, or benefits.

Section 3 — What to Do When Records Are Misleading or False

Not all harmful documentation is factually incorrect in a technical sense. Sometimes, the record reflects what a provider *wrote* — but not what actually happened. These entries may be vague, one-sided, or written in ways that distort your behavior, motives, or credibility. When that happens, the record becomes **misleading**, and you have the right to challenge it under federal law.

According to **5 U.S.C. § 552a(d)** and **38 C.F.R. § 1.579**, you may request correction of **any VA record** that is:

- Inaccurate
- Incomplete
- Irrelevant
- Untimely

This legal standard covers entries that may be technically "factual" (i.e., they were entered by a VA employee) but still **misrepresent or omit the full truth**.

Examples of Misleading or False Entries

- *"Patient refused mental health services."*
  In truth, you asked for a trauma-specific therapist and were denied — not that you refused care.

- *"Patient is noncompliant with treatment."*
  But no one explained the treatment plan, and your decision was medically informed — not defiant.

- *"Veteran was agitated and argumentative during the visit."*
  There is no context for why you were upset — such as being denied access, misunderstood, or provoked.

- *"Patient reports no significant medical issues."*
  The nurse failed to ask the correct intake questions or rushed through the process, and the note misrepresents your responses.

Chapter 13

Why Misleading Entries Matter

These entries:

- Shape how **future providers** treat you
- Influence disability compensation decisions
- Can harm your eligibility for caregiver support, community care, and service-connected benefits

They also undermine **trust** and **credibility** — two things no Veteran should lose because of lazy or biased documentation.

How to Challenge Misleading Documentation

1. Use the Amendment Request Form
   - Describe the entry in detail
   - Explain how it misrepresents or omits key facts
   - Specify what a fair and accurate correction should reflect

2. Attach a Personal Statement
   - Clearly explain what actually occurred
   - Highlight what was left out, mischaracterized, or distorted
   - Keep your tone factual, not emotional — the goal is to be taken seriously

3. Provide Supporting Evidence
   - After Visit Summaries
   - Secure Messages
   - Previous notes or referrals
   - Witness statements (caregivers, family, case workers)

4. Cite VA Policy If Necessary
   - While you don't need to quote the law, you *can* point out that under **38 C.F.R. § 1.579**, you have a legal right to challenge records that are incomplete or misleading

Sample Statement for a Misleading Note

"The progress note dated 05/12/2024 states I 'refused mental health care.' This is misleading. I told the provider I have a trauma history and asked for a referral to a provider trained in MST. I did not refuse care — I requested appropriate care and was denied. I request this entry be amended to reflect the actual discussion, or that the language be removed."

If the VA Denies Your Request

Even if the VA refuses to amend the note, you still have power:

- Submit a Statement of Disagreement
    - This becomes a permanent part of your VA record
    - It must be included in all future disclosures of the disputed entry
- Escalate the issue
    - If the record is defamatory or harmful, and you believe the denial was improper, you may escalate using the steps covered later in this chapter.

Remember: the goal is to create a **written trail** that tells the full story — one that future reviewers, providers, and legal representatives will see.

Section 4 — Boilerplate Denials and How to Fight Them

When you request an amendment to your VA health record, VA policy is unambiguous: the facility must respond in writing, explain the decision, and cite the legal basis for that decision. Yet many Veterans receive generic "boilerplate" denials — prewritten responses that dismiss the request without genuine consideration or any reference to the actual evidence submitted.

These denials are not just unhelpful. In many cases, they **violate federal law and VA policy.**

What VA Policy Requires in a Denial

Per VA Handbook 6300.4, Section 3(e)(5):

> "The VA notice will specify the reason(s) for denying the request, identify the VA regulations or statutes upon which the denial is based."

This requirement is not optional. Any VA response that fails to meet this standard — by giving vague or templated responses with no statutory reference — is procedurally **noncompliant.**

In addition, **38 C.F.R. § 1.579(d)** requires that any denial of a Privacy Act amendment request must:

- Be in writing
- Contain the **specific reason(s)** for the denial
- Inform the Veteran of their right to:
  - Submit a Statement of Disagreement
  - Request a review by the Office of General Counsel

Common Boilerplate Denial Language (and What's Wrong with It)

Some of the most common boilerplate responses Veterans receive include:

- *"The provider stands by their note."*
  → This is not a valid explanation. It fails to engage with your evidence and does not satisfy the requirement to cite a regulatory basis.

- *"Clinical documentation is not subject to change."*
  → Incorrect. VA records *are* subject to change under **5 U.S.C. § 552a(d)** and **VHA Directive 1605.01**, when the record is inaccurate, incomplete, irrelevant, or untimely.

- *"We do not amend records based on patient disagreement."*
  → Misleading and false. The **entire purpose** of a Privacy Act amendment request is to address a patient's disagreement with the contents of a VA record.

- *"We find that the information you requested to be amended is accurate and relevant in its current form."*
  → This conclusory language offers no explanation or evidence. Without citing what was reviewed or which regulation supports the denial, it violates **VA Handbook 6300.4**.

- *"This is a templated question with no ability to make comments."*
  → This response implies that the VA cannot amend the record due to software limitations. That is **not an acceptable justification** for denying a request under federal law.

Chapter 13

How to Respond to a Noncompliant Denial

If you receive a denial that does not meet the clear standards of **Section 3(e)(5)** of VA Handbook 6300.4, take the following steps:

1. Formally Request a Compliant Denial Letter

    Submit a written reply to the Privacy Officer:

    > "*I respectfully request a revised response that complies with VA Handbook 6300.4, Section 3(e)(5), which requires VA to specify the reasons for denial and cite the regulations or statutes that support the decision. The current denial lacks both and does not meet this legal requirement.*"

    This puts the Privacy Officer on notice that **you are aware of your rights** and that you expect a policy-compliant reply.

2. Submit a Statement of Disagreement

    Even if the denial is vague or improper, you still have the right to submit a **Statement of Disagreement**. This statement must become a permanent part of your medical record and must be disclosed alongside the disputed entry anytime that portion of your record is shared. This right is protected under both **38 C.F.R. § 1.579(e)** and **5 U.S.C. § 552a(d)(4)**.

3. File a Complaint for Policy Violation

    If you continue to receive vague or dismissive responses, file a formal complaint under **VHA Directive 1003.04 (Veteran Complaint Management)**. Reference the violation of:

    - VA Handbook 6300.4, Section 3(e)(5)
    - 38 C.F.R. § 1.579(d)
    - Your rights under the Privacy Act (5 U.S.C. § 552a)

    You may also report the issue to the **Patient Advocate, VISN Privacy Officer**, or escalate through the facility's chain of command.

4. Use the Denial as Evidence of Systemic Failure

   If the denial is part of a larger pattern — such as repeated failures to amend false notes, staff retaliating for complaints, or recordkeeping used to undermine benefits — document this. A single improper denial may justify a new amendment request. Multiple denials may justify:

   - A pattern-of-failure complaint to **VISN leadership**
   - A submission to the Office of Inspector General (OIG)
   - A **Congressional inquiry** or legislative advocacy request

Sample Response Letter

Subject: Request for Revised Denial Letter (Amendment Request Dated [Date])

Dear [Privacy Officer Name],

I am writing in response to the denial letter I received concerning my amendment request submitted on [date]. The denial did not specify the reason for the denial or cite the VA regulations or statutes upon which the denial was based.

According to VA Handbook 6300.4, Section 3(e)(5): "The VA notice will specify the reason(s) for denying the request, identify the VA regulations or statutes upon which the denial is based." I respectfully request a revised response that complies with this requirement.

I am also submitting a Statement of Disagreement to be added to my official medical record, as permitted by 38 C.F.R. § 1.579(e).

Respectfully,
[Veteran Name]

If your amendment request is ignored, denied with vague reasoning, or dismissed without proper review, escalation is not only appropriate — it may be necessary. In the next section, we'll walk through when to escalate, how to do it effectively, and which policies support your right to push for correction and accountability.

Section 5 — When to Escalate and How

Veterans don't expect a fight when they request a simple correction to their medical records. But when that request is met with silence, vague denials, or outright defiance of policy, escalation becomes necessary — not just to fix your own record, but to prevent future harm to others.

This section walks you through how to escalate within the VA system when your amendment request is improperly handled, based entirely on your rights under:

- 5 U.S.C. § 552a(d) (Privacy Act of 1974)
- 38 C.F.R. § 1.579
- VA Handbook 6300.4, Section 3(e)(5)
- VHA Directive 1605.01

When Should You Escalate?

Escalation is appropriate if:

- You receive **no acknowledgment** of your request within 10 business days
- You receive a **boilerplate denial** with no specific explanation or no citation to VA law or regulation
- Your request is **ignored or delayed** beyond 30 business days (plus one allowable 30-day extension)
- The denial letter **misstates VA policy** or tells you that records "cannot be changed"
- Your concerns are **dismissed** without reviewing your evidence or supporting documents

Step-by-Step Escalation Process

Step 1 — Re-engage the Privacy Officer

Send a follow-up message or letter citing **VA Handbook 6300.4, Section 3(e)(5)**:

"This response does not meet the VA's required standard for Privacy Act denials. Please provide a revised response that includes the specific reasons for denial and cites the regulations or statutes upon which the decision is based."

Be firm but professional. Give a 7- to 10-day deadline for a compliant response.

Step 2 — Submit a Formal Complaint

If the Privacy Officer does not correct the error or refuses to comply:

- File a complaint with the Patient Advocate under VHA Directive 1003.04 (Veteran Complaint Management).
    - Clearly state that the facility's Privacy Officer failed to comply with federal privacy policy
    - Include a copy of the original request, the denial letter, and your written follow-up
- Emphasize the risk of ongoing harm if the inaccurate or misleading information is not corrected

Step 3 — Escalate to VISN Privacy Leadership

If the local Privacy Officer and Patient Advocate do not resolve the issue:

- Contact the VISN (Veterans Integrated Service Network) Privacy Officer
- Reference your unresolved amendment request and include your documentation trail
- Make it clear you are escalating under federal law and VA-wide policy, not just personal dissatisfaction

Step 4 — Submit a Statement of Disagreement

Even if your amendment is denied, you have the right to be heard:

- Submit a Statement of Disagreement under 38 C.F.R. § 1.579(e)
- This becomes a permanent part of your record and must be disclosed alongside the disputed entry

This statement forces VA staff and any future reader of your record to see your side — in your words, not theirs.

Step 5 — Refer to the VA Office of General Counsel

If you believe the denial was retaliatory, biased, or ignored key facts:

- You may request an administrative review by the Office of General Counsel (OGC)
- This is authorized under VA Handbook 6300.4, Section 3(f)
- The OGC has final authority to determine whether VA policy was followed correctly

Optional: Notify Your Congressional Representative

If you experience a pattern of noncompliance — such as repeated denials, improper recordkeeping, or systemic bias — notify your U.S. Representative or Senator:

- Provide your documentation trail
- Explain how the VA is not following its own regulations
- Request their assistance in holding the facility accountable

Build Your Escalation on Policy — Not Emotion

When escalating, always cite the following:

- **VA Handbook 6300.4, Section 3(e)(5):** requires that denials state reasons and cite the specific regulation

- **38 C.F.R. § 1.579:** provides the right to correct inaccurate, incomplete, irrelevant, or untimely records

- **VHA Directive 1605.01:** outlines the privacy rights and amendment procedures for all VA patients

- **5 U.S.C. § 552a:** the federal Privacy Act under which all other regulations are grounded

You are not asking for a favor. You are asserting a legal right backed by federal statute and VA-wide policy. If the system resists — keep going. Every escalation creates a paper trail. Every paper trail is a warning: **"This Veteran knows the rules — and knows when they're being broken."**

Conclusion: Your Record, Your Rights

VA medical records shape how you're treated, what benefits you receive, and how future clinicians understand your health. When those records are wrong — and you correct them — you're not just protecting your file. You're protecting your future.

This chapter showed you how to assert that right with clarity, precision, and legal backing. You now know how to request an amendment, how to respond to boilerplate denials, and how to escalate when the system refuses to correct its own mistakes.

In the next section, we'll look at the deeper problem: what to do when a record isn't just wrong — it's misleading, defamatory, or written in a way that puts your credibility, care, or benefits at risk.

Chapter 14: Recognizing Hidden Hazards in Your VA Record

What I discovered in my own VA medical record forced me to learn the system — not by choice, but by necessity.

For years, I reviewed every doctor's note in my VA medical record. I always believed in staying informed and making sure what was written matched what actually happened. But there was one part of the record I never thought to check: the nursing intake. I assumed it was just vitals — blood pressure, weight, maybe a quick medication confirmation. Nothing that could affect a diagnosis, delay care, or impact my eligibility for benefits. I couldn't have been more wrong.

It wasn't until years later, after noticing gaps in my care and how I was being perceived by providers, that I discovered what was really going on. With the help of a nurse from one of the national VA support lines, I took a closer look. What she found stunned me. Across four years of primary care visits — documented by three different nurses — the same types of false or misleading entries kept appearing. Statements I never made were documented as fact. Assessments were logged without any basis — or even a single question. And every one of those entries painted a picture of someone far more capable and functional than I actually was — all without anyone asking me a single question.

These entries weren't harmless. They misled specialists, delayed critical diagnoses, and created barriers when I applied for benefits I had clearly earned. They were buried in plain sight, in a part of the record no one ever thought to question.

When I finally tried to correct them, the system pushed back. Nurses denied my amendment requests without explanation. The Privacy Office ignored policies that require detailed denial justifications. The Patient Advocate office refused to step in. The very protections that are supposed to safeguard Veterans were either inactive — or actively discouraging me from continuing.

That experience forced me to learn the rules: the legal standards behind medical documentation, the procedures for amending records, and the actual role of the Patient Advocate. It drove me to help others. And ultimately, it led me to write this book.

This chapter is personal — but it's also practical. I'll walk you through the types of inaccurate entries I found in my own record, explain what they mean, and what should have happened instead — because if they happened to me, they may be happening to you. While this chapter won't revisit how to file an amendment request (covered earlier in the book), it will help you recognize the kinds of charting errors that often go unnoticed and unchallenged.

If it happened to me, it's likely happening to others. And unless you know where to look, you may never know what's been said about you — or how far the damage has spread.

Section 1 — The Nursing Intake: A Hidden Source of Harm

For years, I trusted the system more than I realized. Like many Veterans, I carefully reviewed my doctor's notes after every VA appointment. I looked for accuracy, made sure medications were right, and kept my own records aligned. But one section — the nursing intake — I never thought to check.

I assumed it was just vitals. A quick blood pressure reading. Weight. Maybe a few clicks to verify allergies or meds. But what I didn't realize is that the intake includes much more — and in my case, that "much more" became a serious problem.

It wasn't just one visit. It was four years' worth of routine primary care intakes. Three different nurses. Across all of them, the same types of false, misleading, or outright fabricated entries appeared again and again. They were buried several screens deep in my chart — a place I never had a reason to look. And because I didn't catch them early, they stayed in my record for years.

These entries weren't minor errors. They had consequences:

- They falsely stated I had no changes in daily living or physical function, even during times of major decline.

- They reported that I exercised regularly — despite my condition making that impossible — and no one ever asked me.

- They claimed I said I was "*functioning effectively on my treatment plan,*" when I wasn't even asked the question.

- They stated there were "*no potential barriers to learning,*" even though I had a documented TBI diagnosis with memory loss.

Each of these entries created a version of me that didn't exist. A version who didn't need follow-up care. A version who didn't need accommodation. A version who was healthier, stronger, and more independent than I truly was.

Worse, these false entries confused specialists, influenced decision-making, and delayed diagnoses and treatment I should have received earlier. They didn't just distort my record — they distorted my care.

This section exists to make sure that doesn't happen to you. In the next sections, I'll walk through each of the specific charting errors I found — how they're supposed to be used, how they were misused, and what Veterans should look for in their own records.

Because nursing intake may seem like a formality. But when it's wrong — and no one checks it — it becomes a barrier to the very care you earned.

Section 2 — The Braden Scale: Misused and Misleading

The Braden Scale was never designed for routine outpatient care. It's a tool meant to assess the risk of pressure ulcers in patients who are bedridden, hospitalized, or receiving long-term care — not Veterans walking into a primary care clinic for a scheduled appointment.

Yet in my case, it showed up again and again in the nursing intake documentation. And every time, it was marked as complete — with a perfect score of 23.

On the surface, that might seem harmless. A score of 23 means "low or no risk," and for someone not at risk of pressure ulcers, that might seem accurate. But here's the problem: the assessment should never have been administered in the first place.

The Braden Scale evaluates factors like sensory perception, moisture, activity, mobility, nutrition, and friction/shear. These categories are only meaningful when the patient is in a setting where skin breakdown is a real and present concern. Unless a Veteran has documented immobility, skin issues, or other clear risk factors, there is no clinical justification for using this tool during a quick outpatient intake.

In my case, I had none of the risk factors — but I also wasn't asked about mobility or examined for skin issues. The score of 23 was the result of default answers, likely entered without direct observation. That kind of entry does more than pad the chart — it paints a distorted picture of my health. It creates a clinical suggestion that I am fully mobile, functional, and independent, even when my records elsewhere reflect otherwise.

Used improperly, the Braden Scale doesn't just waste time. It actively misrepresents patients. And when it becomes part of your longitudinal health record — especially over the course of years — it can influence treatment decisions, reduce urgency for referrals, and even affect eligibility for certain benefits tied to mobility or functional status.

This isn't about one form being used the wrong way. It's about a pattern of documentation that can make you look healthier than you are — without anyone realizing it, including you.

Section 3 — "Functioning Effectively on Current Pain Plan" Without Ever Asking

One of the most misleading entries in my VA record wasn't a misdiagnosis — it was a false affirmation:

> **"States IS able to function effectively on the current treatment plan."**

The problem? I never said that.

Worse, no one ever asked. When I later challenged the entry, the nurse acknowledged it wasn't a direct quote, but rather her clinical opinion — documented in a way that made it look like my own words. This subtle misrepresentation suggested that I was stable and improving, when in reality I was in one of the most physically painful and functionally impaired periods of my life.

At that point, I was suffering from severe pain in my neck and shoulder. I couldn't sleep through the night, lie on one side, get out of bed unassisted, or use my dominant arm for basic tasks. I needed my spouse's help to eat, dress, and manage hygiene. My functional capacity had dropped dramatically — and I had already reported these issues to the VA, both verbally and in writing. My symptoms had also been recently documented by another provider, who noted that I was *not* functioning effectively.

No questions were asked about how my pain was impacting daily activities. There was no follow-up about my ability to move, rest, cook, clean, or complete hygiene tasks. And despite written documentation already in the chart that contradicted the "functioning effectively" claim, that misleading phrase was still added.

Compounding the issue was the misuse of the Defense and Veterans Pain Rating Scale (DVPRS) — the VA's standard tool for assessing pain. The DVPRS asks Veterans to rate their pain on a scale from 0 to 10, where each number is linked to how pain affects everyday life: sleeping, eating, working, socializing, and more.

But here's the catch: the DVPRS doesn't indicate whether a score applies to localized pain or overall pain — and most of the time, neither does the nurse entering it into your record. Let's say you go to an appointment for knee pain. The nurse may ask about your knee — not your back, neck, or anything else. If you say your knee pain is a 4 out of 10, and your neck pain is an 8 that keeps you from dressing or sleeping, only the knee score gets recorded. Unless the nurse clearly documents that the score is condition-specific, anyone reading the note may assume the pain score reflects your overall status.

That's exactly what happened to me — repeatedly. Nurses failed to clarify which condition the DVPRS score applied to. Then, they paired it with a default entry stating I was "functioning effectively on the current treatment plan." Together, these entries created a false image: that I was stable and managing well, when I was in rapid decline and barely functioning.

Entries like this may seem small, but they ripple outward. They affect how future providers interpret your condition. They mislead claims evaluators reviewing your medical history. They make it appear that your care plan is working — when in reality, you may be deteriorating.

And if you don't catch it, no one else will.

Always double-check the pain screening and functional status sections. These are not just routine checkboxes — they define how the system sees you. And if they're wrong, they can misrepresent your reality in ways that are hard to undo.

Chapter 14

Section 4 — Dismissal of Documented Cognitive Limitations

One of the most consistently inaccurate statements I found in my medical record appeared in four separate nursing intake assessments — all by different nurses over the course of four years. In each instance, the nurse documented that I had *"no apparent potential barriers to learning."*

That might sound routine, even benign. But it wasn't true.

At the time of these entries, I had a clearly documented diagnosis of traumatic brain injury (TBI) with mild memory loss. That diagnosis wasn't buried — it was backed by a full neuropsychological evaluation conducted by the VA and filed years earlier. Among other findings, the evaluation noted impairments in contextual memory, auditory working memory, delayed recall, and several executive functions essential for learning and processing information. In other words, I had medically documented cognitive limitations. Yet not a single nurse conducting these intakes asked me about them. And not one referenced or acknowledged the existing evaluation.

Had they asked, I would have told them. I've experienced memory lapses that interfere with how I retain and apply information — especially when instructions are verbal, rapid, or only given once. But those questions were never posed. Instead, my record was populated with broad statements declaring that I had no learning barriers — statements that directly contradicted my diagnosis.

When I later submitted an amendment request to have these entries corrected, I was met with resistance. Each nurse defended their note by stating it reflected their clinical assessment based on "multiple interactions" with me — suggesting that their brief subjective impressions during a fast-paced intake somehow overrode the conclusions of a formal neuropsychological evaluation conducted by a trained specialist. Even after I pointed out that this evaluation was in the very record they claimed to have reviewed, the denials stood.

These statements didn't just distort my chart — they misrepresented my capacity, misinformed my providers, and undermined my credibility. They gave the impression that I had no difficulties understanding medical information, complying with treatment, or remembering instructions — when that was far from reality.

Chapter 14

This is exactly why it's so important to review even the most routine-seeming parts of your medical record. Inaccuracies like this can go unchecked for years, repeated visit after visit, and no one will notice — unless you do.

Section 5: Failure to Document Changes in Activities of Daily Living (ADLs)

Another critical intake error in my VA record was the failure to acknowledge significant changes in my activities of daily living (ADLs) — particularly those related to mobility, personal hygiene, dressing, and eating — during a time when I was experiencing acute pain and functional impairment.

Despite clear evidence in my chart and my verbal communication at the time, the intake nurse marked "No" to the question: *"Have there been any changes in your activities of daily living in the past 30 days?"*

In reality, my ability to perform ADLs had declined sharply. Due to severe pain in my neck and right shoulder, I was unable to lie on my right side, roll over without assistance, or get out of bed on my own. I required my spouse's help with nearly every aspect of daily life. I couldn't use my dominant arm to feed myself, dress, or manage hygiene. After using the restroom, I needed help cleaning myself. I couldn't button shirts, pull on pants, or even undress without assistance. These were all new and serious limitations, and they occurred within the exact 30-day window the intake form asked about.

The nurse conducting the intake did not ask about ADLs at all. As a result, these changes went undocumented. Compounding the issue, I had already reported the severity of my condition days earlier in a secure message, and another provider had recently documented that I was *"not able to function effectively on the current treatment plan."* That same provider also noted that my pain had an intensity of 7–8 out of 10 and was aggravated by basic movements like lifting my arm or turning my head.

Even though this context was readily available in my record — and even though I had reiterated it in writing and over the phone — the intake nurse marked "No" for ADL changes. That simple click of a box created the false impression that I was still functioning normally and independently.

This wasn't a one-time issue. It happened during a period of obvious decline, at a time when I was being referred to urgent care, prescribed high-dose medications, and struggling to get through the day. Failing to ask about — or accurately document — changes in ADLs during a time like this is not just an oversight. It's a misrepresentation of the patient's condition and a missed opportunity to ensure the care team is fully informed.

Statements about ADLs matter. They influence eligibility for caregiver support, disability evaluations, referrals for rehabilitation, and even pain management options. A "No" answer when the real answer is "Yes" can delay or deny critical services. And unless patients actively challenge those entries, they stand uncontested — misleading everyone who reads them afterward.

Section 6: False Reporting of Physical Activity

Across multiple VA intake encounters, nurses consistently recorded that I exercise for at least 30 minutes, three times per week. This statement was entered as if it were fact — despite the reality that I am physically incapable of engaging in any kind of structured exercise routine due to longstanding medical limitations.

At no point during these visits was I asked about my ability to exercise. The intake nurses simply selected a default or assumed answer. This resulted in false entries that painted a misleading picture of my physical condition, one that directly contradicted dozens of clinical notes in my VA record.

For years, my medical history has documented my inability to exercise due to serious physical impairments. These limitations were not subtle. They were well-documented by primary care providers, specialists, and physical therapists across dozens of visits. In multiple notes, providers explicitly wrote "unable to exercise" or "does not exercise due to symptoms." My records show repeated and consistent evidence of exertional symptoms, physical deconditioning, and emergency care triggered by mild activity.

Despite all of this, the intake nurses continued to document that I was physically active. This kind of documentation does more than just obscure the truth — it risks influencing future care decisions, such as eligibility for home-based care, caregiver support, and service connection increases. It can also delay referrals or cause clinicians to assume that I am managing better than I truly am.

Even when I brought these errors to the attention of the nurse involved, she defended her documentation rather than acknowledge the discrepancy. Rather than advocate for accuracy or update the record to reflect my functional reality, her concern appeared to be justifying her prior entry — not patient care.

One of the most concerning examples involved an intake nurse referencing a specialist's note to justify an amendment denial for her false exercise documentation. She selectively quoted a sentence suggesting I was "active," but ignored the very sentence preceding it, which stated: "The patient does not perform all activities of daily living without restriction." She also omitted critical context that clearly contradicted her implication that I was physically active.

This kind of cherry-picking — whether intentional or negligent — misrepresents the complexity of a patient's condition. It reflects a deeper problem: when VA staff fail to review a Veteran's chart or engage in honest, thorough questioning, they risk embedding falsehoods into the medical record. And once those entries are made, they are treated as clinical fact — unless the Veteran challenges them.

These kinds of statements are not harmless. They can derail treatment planning, mislead benefits evaluators, and result in clinical decisions that are based on a fictional version of the patient's health. And unless Veterans actively correct them, they stay in the system — unchallenged and deeply consequential.

Conclusion — Don't Let the Record Rewrite Your Reality

What I've shared in this chapter isn't just my story — it's a warning. These kinds of charting errors are happening to Veterans across the country, often without their knowledge. Most of us never think to check the nursing intake. We assume it's just vitals or harmless screening questions. But what gets documented — or misdocumented — becomes clinical fact. It shapes how doctors view us, how referrals are prioritized, how benefits are evaluated, and how the system decides what kind of care we "need."

Inaccurate records don't just distort the past — they can derail your future. They influence diagnoses, delay treatment, undermine claims, and misrepresent your capacity at every level. And once those entries are made, they echo forward in ways that are hard to undo.

You have a right to see your full medical record — and a responsibility to protect it. Read every section, especially the ones no one talks about. Question what doesn't match your experience. And when you find something wrong, don't let it stand.

You're not being difficult. You're defending your truth — and in a system that often values process over people, that's how you stay visible, credible, and in control.

PART V

Support Systems and Coordinated Care

> *"When the system works, it works together — but sometimes, you have to remind it how."*

The VA health care system isn't just doctors and appointments — it's social workers, Whole Health teams, caregiver programs, home-based care, and coordinated services that are supposed to support you beyond the clinic walls.

But here's the problem: many Veterans never get connected to these resources. Others are denied access outright — often because their records are inaccurate, their needs are misunderstood, or their conditions don't fit neatly into checkboxes.

This section is about bringing it all together:

- How VA social workers can and should advocate for you when care falls apart
- What the Whole Health program is — and how to use it to rebuild your quality of life
- How PACT teams are supposed to coordinate care — and what to do when they don't
- What you can do when you're told, *"We don't offer that here"* — even when VA policy says otherwise

These chapters will help you access the support systems that too often go unused or underused. If you've ever felt like no one was looking at the full picture — or that your care was fragmented and reactive — this is where you learn how to change that.

Because real care isn't just about treating symptoms. It's about recognizing the person behind the diagnosis — and making the system work together for the life you're still trying to live.

Chapter 15: Using Social Work for Advocacy and Support

When your care breaks down, you're not supposed to be alone in fixing it. VA social workers are trained, licensed professionals with a mandate to advocate for you—not just in theory, but according to formal policy. **VHA Directive 1110.02** lays out in clear language that VA social work services are a core part of the health care system, and that every Veteran has the right to receive support for navigating complex care needs, community resources, and systemic barriers. These aren't just helpers—they're supposed to be your frontline defenders when the system fails to deliver.

This chapter breaks down that policy and shows you how to use it. You'll learn what social workers are supposed to do, when to ask for one, and how to respond when they ignore their responsibilities. Because advocacy isn't your burden to carry alone. The VA created a role for that. It's time to hold them to it.

Section 1 — The Role of VA Social Workers: More Than Case Managers

Most Veterans think of social workers as people who help with housing or mental health referrals. But within the VA, their role is far broader—and far more powerful—than many realize. According to VHA Directive 1110.02, VA social workers are master's-level, licensed professionals who are embedded throughout nearly every clinical care setting in the Veterans Health Administration. They are not just case managers—they are care coordinators, resource specialists, crisis responders, and most importantly, advocates.

The directive makes their responsibility to advocate unmistakably clear. It states:

> "*The VA medical facility social worker is responsible for Providing Client advocacy AND Advocating for eligible Service members, Veterans, their families, and caregivers when they experience challenges in meeting their health care needs.*" (Sections 2(p)(1)(n) & 2(p)(1)(t)).

This means that when a Veteran's access to care is delayed, when services are denied, or when VA staff are unresponsive, the social worker is not just allowed to intervene—they are required to**.** Advocacy is not something they do "on the side"; it is a defined, clinical responsibility under VA policy.

Their role includes conducting psychosocial assessments, developing individualized care plans, supporting transitions of care, and coordinating services both inside and outside the VA. But beyond those functions, social workers are expected to act when other parts of the system fail. If a Veteran isn't getting the care they need because of poor communication, bureaucratic delays, or systemic gaps, the social worker is the one who should step forward.

This is why understanding their role matters. VA social workers aren't optional helpers—they are assigned allies with a mandate to act. And when they don't, it's not just disappointing. It's a breach of policy, and one that can and should be challenged.

Section 2 — How to Ask for a Social Worker — and What to Expect

You don't need a referral or an emergency to speak with a VA social worker. If you're facing care delays, referral breakdowns, trouble coordinating outside services, or any health-related issue that isn't being addressed through your provider, you have the right to request social work support directly.

Here are different ways to request a social worker:

- **Tell your PACT team or front desk**: Ask, "Can I speak with a social worker about care coordination?" You don't need to give full details up front.

- **Use Secure Messaging** through MyHealtheVet: Send a message to your care team with the subject line, "Request for Social Work Assistance."

- **Call the main facility line**: Ask for "Social Work Services" or the "Social Work Department."

- **During appointments**, tell your nurse or provider: "I need help coordinating services — could someone from Social Work reach out to me?"

Every VA facility is staffed with licensed social workers, and each PACT team has access to one. Don't let anyone tell you they're not available.

Chapter 15

What to Expect:

- Most social workers will contact you within a few business days.
- They may offer a phone call, video visit, or in-person appointment.
- The first step is often a **psychosocial assessment**, which helps identify what barriers you're facing and how they can help.

What If You're Blocked or Dismissed?

Some Veterans are incorrectly told:

- *"You need to speak with your provider first."*
- *"They only handle discharges."*
- *"That's not something social work helps with."*
- *"They're not available today."*

If this happens, respond with:

"Can you connect me with the Social Work supervisor?"

"If no one is available, I'd like to leave a message or send a Secure Message directly."

Keep a record of who you spoke to and what they said. If needed, escalate through the Patient Advocate Office, or file a formal request for social work intervention.

Use Clear, Specific Language

Being vague can result in your request being deprioritized or misunderstood. Try phrases like:

- *"My care coordination has broken down and I need help."*
- *"A referral has been delayed, and no one is returning my messages."*
- *"I'm dealing with multiple conditions and falling through the cracks."*
- *"I'm not getting answers, and I'd like a social worker to get involved."*

Social workers are trained to assist in these exact situations — but you may have to advocate for access.

If You're Still Blocked

If a staff member refuses to refer you or says "that's not their job," take these steps:

1. Ask who supervises Social Work Services at the facility.
2. Send a Secure Message documenting your request and what happened.
3. Contact the Patient Advocate Office and include the name of the person who blocked access.
4. Consider escalating as described in Chapter 8.

Getting access to the help you need shouldn't be this hard — but when it is, you're not asking for special treatment. You're asking the VA to follow its own policy and provide the support it already promises.

Section 3 — Common Situations That Require Social Work Intervention

VA social workers are not just there for discharge planning or referrals — they are trained to intervene when a Veteran's access to care, safety, or coordination falls apart. The following are some of the most common (and often overlooked) scenarios where social work assistance is not only appropriate but essential.

1. Missed or Delayed Referrals

If your referral was placed but never scheduled — or the clinic tells you they never received it — this is a breakdown in coordination. A social worker can trace the referral path, identify where it stalled, and push the request forward. They can also document the delay and ensure your provider is alerted.

2. Communication Failures Between Clinics or Providers

When your primary care provider says one thing, and your specialist says another — or when no one is responding at all — a social worker can act as a bridge. They're trained to collaborate across departments, resolve handoff issues, and bring clarity to tangled lines of communication.

3. Social Drivers of Health (SDOH)

If housing instability, food insecurity, caregiving responsibilities, or financial barriers are affecting your health or access to care, these are considered SDOH factors — and they are directly within the scope of social work intervention under VHA Directive 1110.02. You don't have to fix these things alone. In fact, you're not supposed to.

4. Discharge Without Aftercare or Coordination

If you're released from inpatient care with no follow-up plan, or your aftercare instructions are unclear, a social worker can help coordinate next steps, verify follow-up appointments, and ensure continuity of care. This includes mental health discharges, which can be especially vulnerable to gaps.

5. Family, Caregiver, or Survivor Struggles

If a spouse, caregiver, or surviving family member is trying to navigate the system on your behalf — or is overwhelmed due to your condition — social workers are authorized to intervene and support both you and your support team. This includes helping with caregiver eligibility, respite coordination, or grief counseling referrals.

6. Transportation or Access Barriers

If you're missing appointments because of travel limitations, live in a rural area, or don't qualify for travel pay but still need support, this is a situation where a social worker may be able to coordinate Community Care, home visits, or outreach to non-VA partners.

7. Being Told *"There's Nothing More We Can Do"*

If you've hit a wall with your care team and are told "there's nothing more we can do" — and you know that's not true — it's time to involve a social worker. They can review your case and help determine what options still exist, including second opinions, consults at other VA facilities, or a formal review by leadership.

8. Complex or Chronic Conditions Needing Coordinated Support

Veterans dealing with multiple diagnoses or chronic illness often face uncoordinated treatment across specialties. This is a textbook case for social work involvement. They are trained to handle complex coordination, case management, and care planning that goes beyond any one provider's scope.

In all these situations, the VA's own policy makes clear: social workers have the clinical authority and responsibility to step in. If your situation matches one of these patterns and no one is offering help — you're not being difficult. You're being underserved.

Section 4 — What to Do When a Social Worker Doesn't Help?

Even though VA social workers are required to advocate for you and help resolve care challenges, some fail to follow through. If you're met with silence, deflection, or a flat refusal to help, you're not out of options — you're just at the beginning of a different kind of advocacy.

Recognize the Problem

You should expect a response within days, a clear effort to assess your needs, and meaningful follow-up. If you're being ignored or dismissed and the issue remains unresolved, this likely reflects a breakdown in the VA's duty to provide client advocacy under VHA Directive 1110.02.

Document the Interaction

Keep track of who you contacted, when you contacted them, what you asked for, and what response (if any) you received. This is your complaint log — a key part of your paper trail if the issue needs to be escalated.

Follow Up Respectfully

If a social worker's response was vague, inadequate, or delayed, send a polite but clear message:

> *"I'm following up on my previous request for social work assistance. My issue remains unresolved, and I would appreciate timely support coordinating care."*

Putting this in writing — especially through Secure Messaging — reinforces that you've made a reasonable effort.

Escalate to Supervisors

If you're still not getting help, ask for the Supervisory Social Worker or Chief of Social Work Service. Be direct, and cite VHA Directive 1110.02, which requires social workers to advocate for Veterans experiencing challenges accessing health care.

Submit a Formal Complaint

If internal escalation fails, file a complaint through the Patient Advocate, the Facility Director, or the VA Office of Inspector General (OIG). Include dates, names, summaries of each interaction, and references to the directive. A clear, documented failure to assist strengthens your case.

Keep the Goal in Sight

You're not doing this to get someone in trouble — you're trying to fix a gap in care. A working social work team can help you navigate complex systems, link services, and protect your health and well-being. If you push for accountability, it's because you're protecting your access to that support.

Section 5 — When to Escalate and How

If you've followed up, documented your concerns, and still haven't received appropriate support from a VA social worker, it's time to escalate.

Start with the Supervisory Social Worker or the Chief of Social Work Service at your facility. These leaders are responsible for ensuring that social workers follow the requirements in VHA Directive 1110.02, including providing client advocacy and coordinating care when Veterans face challenges accessing services.

If that step fails, you can file a complaint with:

- The Patient Advocate Office
- The Facility Director
- The VA Office of Inspector General (OIG) if systemic neglect or misconduct is suspected

In your complaint, be specific. Describe the issue, provide a timeline, and cite the relevant sections of the directive:

> "The VA medical facility social worker is responsible for providing client advocacy and advocating for eligible Service members, Veterans, their families, and caregivers when they experience challenges in meeting their health care needs."
> (VHA Directive 1110.02, Sections 2(p)(1)(n) & (t))

For templates, escalation steps, and follow-up tracking tools, refer to Chapters 7 and 8. These tools work no matter which VA service line is failing you — and that includes social work.

Social workers are more than just referral sources — they are trained, accountable professionals with a defined responsibility to advocate for you, especially when the VA care system breaks down. VHA Directive 1110.02 makes this clear: when you are facing chronic illness, complex needs, or gaps in care, social workers are required to step in.

But as you've seen, that doesn't always happen. When it doesn't, your job is to document, follow up, and escalate — not just for yourself, but for every Veteran who deserves better.

When you assert your right to competent, engaged social work support, you are not asking for favors. You are demanding that the system function as promised — with dignity, accountability, and professionalism.

And when the system doesn't deliver, you now know how to respond.

In the chapters that follow, we'll look at other programs and team structures — like Whole Health and PACT — that are designed to support your care across VA silos.

Chapter 16: Exploring Whole Health and Veteran Empowerment

What matters to you should shape the care you receive — not just what's the matter with you. That's the core principle behind the VA's Whole Health System of Care, a nationally mandated model that places your values, goals, and life priorities at the center of your treatment.

This isn't a pilot program or a wellness trend. Under VHA Directive 1445, every VA medical center is required to implement Whole Health as a core part of the standard medical benefits package. This system includes three foundational components:

- **Veteran-centered Personal Health Planning** — structured conversations that help you define what matters most and create a personalized plan of care.

- **Well-being Programs** — resources and services that support your health goals, such as mindfulness, tai chi, nutrition, movement, and stress reduction.

- **Whole Health Clinical Care** — integration of your goals and values into your traditional treatment plan, delivered through a team-based model.

If you've never been offered these services — or were told they weren't available at your facility — you're not alone. Many VA staff remain unfamiliar with the directive's requirements or treat Whole Health as optional. But it's not. It's a formal policy with clear implementation standards and assigned responsibilities.

This chapter gives you the tools to access these services, advocate for your right to personalized care, and hold VA leadership accountable when the system falls short. Whether you're just starting out or already hitting roadblocks, what follows will help you shift from passive patient to empowered partner in your own health journey.

Section 1 — What the Whole Health System Really Is (and What It Isn't)

If you've heard of "Whole Health" at the VA, it may have been in the context of a yoga class, a mindfulness session, or an optional support group. Unfortunately, many Veterans are introduced to it this way — as a supplemental service, loosely tied to wellness but not central to their care.

But that's not how the VA defines it.

1. **Veteran-Centered Personal Health Planning**
   Veterans must have the opportunity to participate in developing a personal health plan (PHP) that reflects what matters most to them, with a structured process for goal-setting and follow-up.

2. **Well-Being Programs**
   These offer activities that support lifestyle, resilience, and personal health goals. They may include group classes or services like meditation, movement therapies, or other self-care education.

3. **Whole Health Clinical Care**
   VA care teams are expected to integrate Whole Health principles into treatment planning. This includes incorporating CIH therapies and honoring personal health goals as part of ongoing care.

These components are not standalone services. They are integrated into how your VA care should be delivered — tailored to your needs, informed by your goals, and reinforced through both primary care and specialty services.

Yet many facilities are behind in implementation. Some VA staff may not even be aware of what the directive requires. This disconnect creates confusion and leads Veterans to believe these services are optional, unavailable, or irrelevant. That confusion isn't your fault — but knowing the truth gives you power.

Whole Health is not limited by age, era of service, or diagnosis. It is not reserved for post-9/11 Veterans or only available in certain clinics. It is required by VA policy. When facilities fail to inform you, refer you, or deliver care consistent with this model, they are not just being dismissive — they may be out of compliance.

This section sets the foundation. In the next, you'll learn exactly what services you're entitled to, how to ask for them, and what to do when your facility falls short.

Section 2 — What Services You're Entitled To

The VA's Whole Health System (WHS) is not an optional wellness initiative — it is a mandated model of care that every VA medical facility is required to implement. According to Section 3.c of VHA Directive 1445, all VA facilities must offer specific services and programs designed to help Veterans take charge of their health, driven by their personal goals and values.

1. **Veteran-Centered Whole Health Pathway**
   As outlined in Section 3.c(1), VA facilities must provide access to services that help you explore what matters most to you in life and health. These services are typically delivered by trained Whole Health Partners, Whole Health Coaches, and peers who guide you through the process of reflection, goal setting, and developing a Personal Health Plan. You should be invited to engage in this process, not simply handed a form.

2. **Well-Being Programming**
   Under Section 3.c(2), facilities are required to offer a range of well-being programs. These may include support for movement and exercise, nutrition, mindfulness, yoga, tai chi, stress management, or other complementary approaches. These services must be available as part of your standard VA health benefits, in accordance with 38 C.F.R. § 17.38.

3. **Whole Health Clinical Care**
   Also under Section 3.c(3), clinical care must reflect your personal goals and priorities. That means your provider is expected to integrate your Whole Health Plan into your primary care, mental health care, and specialty treatment. Clinical decisions should reflect not just your medical history, but also what matters most to you.

What This Means for You

If you've never been invited to create a Personal Health Plan, meet with a Whole Health Coach, or attend well-being programming, that doesn't mean you aren't eligible. It may simply mean your facility has not fully implemented its responsibilities under VHA Directive 1445. In that case, you have the right to request those services and reference the directive by name — specifically Section 3.c — when doing so.

The next section will walk you through how to make those requests, track them, and respond effectively when you face confusion, delay, or denial.

Section 3 — How to Ask for These Services

The services outlined in VHA Directive 1445 are not optional add-ons. They are required elements of the VA's Whole Health System, and every Veteran enrolled in VA care has the right to request them. Unfortunately, many Veterans have never been told about Whole Health — and some VA staff may not fully understand or implement the directive.

Here's how to professionally and effectively request Whole Health services while making sure your request is documented and tied to policy.

1. Start with Your PACT Team or Primary Care Provider

Your Primary Care Team (PACT) is your first point of contact for accessing Whole Health. You can say something like:

> *"I would like to be referred to the Whole Health Pathway to begin building my Personal Health Plan. This is a service required by VHA Directive 1445, Section 3.c(1)."*

You may also ask about:

- Speaking with a Whole Health Coach
- Being connected to Whole Health Partners or peers
- Accessing **well-being programs** like tai chi, mindfulness, or healthy cooking classes

2. Request a Referral to the Facility Whole Health Program

Every VA medical center must have a Whole Health Program. If your PACT team is unfamiliar with the details, ask for a referral or contact directly:

> *"Can you refer me to the Whole Health Program Coordinator or Whole Health team at this facility? I'm requesting services required under VHA Directive 1445."*

If you're not sure who to contact, use Secure Messaging to reach the Patient Advocate or Whole Health Point of Contact at your facility.

3. Document Your Request in Secure Messaging or MyHealtheVet

Any formal request for care should be documented. Use MyHealtheVet Secure Messaging to send your request to your care team or provider, and save a copy of the message. Include:

- The date of your request
- Specific services you are asking for (e.g., Whole Health Coach, well-being classes)
- Mention of VHA Directive 1445, particularly Section 3.c(1)-(3)

Example language:

"I am requesting access to Whole Health Pathway services as outlined in VHA Directive 1445. I would like to meet with a Whole Health Coach and begin developing a Personal Health Plan."

4. Follow Up and Escalate When Necessary

If you don't receive a timely or appropriate response:

- Follow up within 7–10 business days
- Forward your request to the Patient Advocate
- Keep track of your messages and any responses in a complaint log (see Appendix E)

If you are told the service is not unavailable or offered, you can respond:

"According to VHA Directive 1445, Section 3.c, all VA medical facilities are required to provide these services. Can you help me find someone at this facility who oversees Whole Health implementation?"

5. Avoid Passive Denials

Sometimes, the barrier isn't a formal denial — it's silence or confusion. A provider may say they're unfamiliar with Whole Health or that they'll "look into it" but never follow up. That's why it's important to:

- Reference policy clearly
- Keep written proof of your requests
- Know your escalation options if the system stalls

The next section will walk you through how to respond when your local VA does not offer the services required by this directive. You'll learn how to escalate appropriately — and use VHA policy as leverage to get the care you're entitled to.

Section 4 — When Services Are Missing, Delayed, or Denied?

You've made the request. You cited the directive. But the system still isn't delivering what's required.

Whether you're told "we don't offer that here," you're placed on a never-ending waitlist, or you simply get ignored — your response needs to be calm, clear, and grounded in policy. VHA Directive 1445 requires every VA medical facility to implement the Whole Health System. That includes you.

Here's how to respond when services are missing, delayed, or denied.

1. Clarify Whether the Response Is a Denial or a Delay

Ask directly:

> "Can you clarify whether I've been denied Whole Health services or if I'm still on a waitlist?"

If it's a denial — even an informal one — request that the response be put in writing or documented in your record.

If it's a delay, ask:

- What the current wait time is
- When you should expect follow-up
- If there is a point of contact for the Whole Health Program at your facility

2. Reference the Directive in Your Follow-Up

Quote Section 3.c of VHA Directive 1445 in writing, such as through Secure Messaging or a follow-up email. Here's sample language:

> "Under VHA Directive 1445, Section 3.c, VA medical facilities are required to offer access to Whole Health Pathway services, well-being programming, and clinical care that aligns with the Whole Health model. I am requesting to be connected with these services as outlined in the directive. Please advise who I can speak to directly about this."

Be polite, direct, and specific. Attach a PDF of the directive if needed.

3. Escalate Within the Facility

If your request continues to be ignored or delayed:

- Contact the Patient Advocate Office
- Ask to speak with the Whole Health Program Coordinator
- Include a copy of your written request and the directive citation

Let them know this is a policy compliance issue, not just a scheduling preference.

4. Use the Chain of Command If Needed

If internal escalation fails, move up:

- Contact the VISN Whole Health Point of Contact
- Submit a written complaint through the Director's Office
- Include a timeline of your requests, referencing dates and responses
- Reference the directive and emphasize that failure to provide these services violates VA policy

You can use Chapter 9 of this book to help structure your formal complaint.

5. Know What the Directive Requires

Section 3.c requires your VA facility to provide:

- **Whole Health Pathway** access (e.g., Whole Health Coaches and Partners)
- **Well-being programs** tied to your goals and interests
- **Clinical care** that reflects your Personal Health Plan and priorities

If you're being told otherwise, you're not wrong — the system is simply out of compliance.

6. Track and Document Every Step

Keep:

- Copies of all your Secure Messages or emails
- Notes from phone calls, including names and dates
- All written responses (even brief ones)
- A copy of VHA Directive 1445 with your key sections highlighted

As with any advocacy, your paper trail is your power.

The final section of this chapter shows you how to use the Whole Health model not just as a service — but as a framework for reclaiming control over your care, your decisions, and your health journey within the VA system.

Section 5 — How to Use the Whole Health System to Take Charge of Your Care

The Whole Health System isn't just about classes or coaching. It's about changing how care is delivered — and how you, the Veteran, are treated within that system. You are not just a diagnosis. You are not a checklist of medications. Whole Health is meant to center your care on what matters most to you.

But like many VA policies, Whole Health works only if you know how to activate it — and insist on it when others overlook or delay it.

1. Start With the "Circle of Health"

The Whole Health approach begins with what VA calls the "Circle of Health." It places **you**, not your condition, at the center.

Ask yourself:

- What do I want my health for?
- What matters most to me — not just medically, but in life?

This is your foundation. When you meet with a Whole Health Coach or begin creating your Personal Health Plan, you'll use these answers to build goals, choose services, and prioritize care decisions.

Chapter 16

2. Request a Personal Health Plan (PHP)

Your Personal Health Plan is more than a worksheet. It's a formal, documented part of your VA care that helps guide your providers and support teams.

You can say:

"I would like to work with someone to create a Personal Health Plan. This is part of the Whole Health Pathway required under VHA Directive 1445, Section 3.c(1)."

This plan should reflect:

- Your life goals and values
- Areas of self-care and interest
- Clinical care aligned with your preferences

It belongs in your record — and it should be referenced during your appointments.

3. Engage in Well-Being Programs That Fit Your Needs

Under the directive, VA facilities are required to offer well-being programs (see Section 3.c(2)). These may include:

- Movement classes like tai chi, yoga, or walking groups
- Nutrition workshops or healthy cooking demos
- Mindfulness or stress-reduction sessions
- Support circles or peer groups

If the options are limited, ask when more are being added — and let your provider know what you're interested in. Your input matters.

4. Expect Your Providers to Align with Whole Health

Whole Health doesn't just happen in coaching sessions — it should shape how your VA providers work with you. According to Section 3.c(3) of the directive, clinical care should align with your Personal Health Plan.

That means:

- Shared decision-making in medical discussions
- Consideration of your goals when planning treatments
- Respect for your autonomy and values

If you're feeling sidelined in your own care, bring the conversation back to your PHP and the Whole Health model. Ask:

> "Can we revisit how this recommendation supports my Whole Health goals?"

5. You Are the Driver. The VA Is the Support System.

Whole Health only works if you're empowered to lead your care. VA staff are there to support your journey — not control it. If they're unfamiliar with Whole Health, share the directive. If they dismiss it, escalate. And if they comply, thank them — and use that opening to go deeper.

Whole Health gives you the framework, language, and policy backing to say:

> "This is my life. This is my care. And I expect the VA to treat it that way."

Whole Health is more than a buzzword. It's a structural shift — backed by policy, mandated by leadership, and promised to every Veteran. But like many reforms in the VA system, it doesn't reach every facility, every clinic, or every Veteran equally. And when that promise breaks down, it's not because the policy doesn't exist. It's because someone didn't follow it.

This chapter showed you how to request services under VHA Directive 1445, how to escalate when they're denied, and how to use the Whole Health model to center your care around what matters most to you — not just what's wrong with you.

You've now seen how Personal Health Planning, well-being programs, and clinician accountability are meant to work together. And more importantly, you've seen how to hold your VA facility accountable when they fall short.

Because when you combine knowledge of the system with the power to demand compliance, you're not just navigating the VA — you're reshaping it. One record, one complaint, one policy citation at a time.

But for Whole Health to truly work, your core care team has to be aligned — which is where PACT coordination becomes critical.

Chapter 17: Navigating Care with Your PACT Team

At the heart of the VA's healthcare system is a promise: that every Veteran enrolled in VA health care will be assigned a stable, coordinated, and patient-centered team — their Patient Aligned Care Team, or PACT. This isn't just a helpful idea. It's a formal model outlined in VHA Handbook 1101.10(2) and backed by federal law under 38 U.S.C. § 7301 and 7311 and 38 C.F.R. § 17.38, which defines what care the VA is legally required to provide.

Your PACT team is supposed to include your primary care provider, a registered nurse, a licensed practical nurse or health technician, and a clerk — all working together with you at the center. The model emphasizes continuity, access, coordination, and respect — but as many Veterans know, this promise can break down. Providers may be reassigned without notice, follow-up delayed, or access to timely care disrupted.

This chapter is your guide to what the PACT model actually requires, how it's supposed to function, and what you can do when it doesn't. You'll learn how to recognize when your rights under the PACT Handbook are being violated, how to request corrections, and how to file a complaint when necessary.

Because when the VA makes continuity of care part of the legal medical benefits package, and then fails to deliver it, that's not just a bad experience — it's a breakdown in compliance. And you have every right to call it out.

Section 1 — What the PACT Handbook Actually Requires

The Patient Aligned Care Team (PACT) model is more than just a buzzword. It is a structured, policy-driven framework defined by **VHA Handbook 1101.10(2)** to ensure that every Veteran receives coordinated, consistent, and proactive primary care. This handbook is not optional guidance — it is a national standard that every VA medical center is required to implement.

Core Team Structure

Every Veteran enrolled in VA primary care must be assigned to a PACT teamlet that includes:

- A **Primary Care Provider (PCP)** — physician, nurse practitioner, or physician assistant

- A **Registered Nurse (RN)** care manager

- A **Clinical Associate** — typically a licensed practical nurse (LPN), medical assistant, or health technician

- A **Clerical Associate** — provides administrative and scheduling support

These individuals are expected to function as a cohesive, collaborative unit, with you — the Veteran — at the center of decision-making.

Continuity and Panel Management

One of the most important requirements of the PACT model is continuity — maintaining a consistent relationship between the Veteran and the care team. According to the Handbook, continuity is essential for:

- Building trust between the Veteran and provider

- Improving outcomes for chronic and preventive care

- Reducing fragmentation and unnecessary care delays

Your assigned provider should not change frequently. When reassignment is necessary, the facility must ensure a smooth transition and inform the Veteran.

The directive also emphasizes panel management — the proactive coordination of care across all Veterans assigned to a team. Teams are required to use clinical reminders, secure messaging, population health tools, and chronic disease registries to ensure that no Veteran falls through the cracks.

Same-Day Access and Proactive Care

The PACT model is also very clear about access to timely care. As stated in Section 8(d)(6) of the Handbook:

> "All PCPs and RNs must ensure they have same-day access (unless it is too late in the day as determined by the individual facility) for face-to-face encounters, telephone encounters and, when required by VHA guidance or policy, other types of encounters."

This is not a suggestion — it is a direct operational requirement. Veterans must be able to reach their PACT team and receive care on the same day for urgent concerns, unless it's legitimately too late in the day to do so. The method of encounter — in-person, telephone, or secure message — must follow current VHA guidance.

The directive goes even further. In **Section 8(d)(8)**, the VA lays out a clear **hierarchy** for managing requests for non-emergency and same-day care. This is designed to **protect continuity of care** — the core of the PACT model:

> Processes for managing patients' requests for non-emergency care and same-day access must implement the principle of continuity of care by preferentially directing requests for nonemergency care according to the following descending hierarchy of care providers**:**
>
> (a) The patient's assigned PCP and other assigned PACT staff;
>
> (b) The designated covering PCP and covering PACT staff;
>
> (c) Any PCP and any PACT staff; and
>
> (d) Next day appointment (if acceptable to the patient) with the patient's assigned or designated covering PCP and other PACT staff.

This means that the VA **must try to route you to your regular provider and care team first**, not just anyone available. If your team is unavailable, the next best option is their designated covering staff. This hierarchy is not just thoughtful — it is **mandatory**. If you're always being sent to random providers or walk-ins without explanation, your care is not being managed according to policy.

By requiring both same-day responsiveness and team-based continuity, the PACT model ensures that Veterans receive **not only fast care — but the right care, from the right people**.

Chapter 17

The Veteran as a Full Team Member

> The handbook emphasizes that you are not a passive recipient of care — you are an active participant. The team is required to respect your values, preferences, and goals. Shared decision-making is not optional.

In short, PACT is designed to provide personalized, proactive, and patient-driven care — not generic, impersonal service. And when that doesn't happen, the system is out of compliance.

Section 2 — When the Team Breaks Down

Despite what the PACT Handbook requires, many Veterans find themselves facing a very different reality: providers constantly change, follow-up care slips through the cracks, and urgent concerns are met with delays or confusion. When this happens, it's not just frustrating — it's a clear failure to meet the standards outlined in VHA Handbook 1101.10(2) and 38 C.F.R. § 17.38, which defines continuity of care and access as guaranteed medical benefits.

Signs Your PACT Team Is Out of Compliance

Here are common examples that indicate a breakdown in the PACT model:

- You're assigned a new primary care provider with no notice or explanation.
- You can't reach your PACT team by phone, secure message, or appointment — even for urgent concerns.
- The same-day access requirement is routinely ignored or substituted with referrals to walk-in clinics.
- Your team fails to coordinate follow-up for test results, referrals, or medication management.
- You're bounced between providers, often repeating your history with no continuity of care.
- Important preventive care (e.g., labs, screenings) is missed due to poor panel management.

These are not isolated administrative issues — they represent policy-level failures.

Why These Failures Matter

The PACT Handbook is clear: continuity, same-day access, and coordinated care are not optional services — they are foundational VA responsibilities. When those responsibilities are routinely neglected, Veterans face higher risks of poor outcomes, delayed diagnoses, worsening chronic conditions, and unnecessary emergency visits.

Moreover, these failures often contribute to deeper frustrations and distrust in the VA system. Many Veterans begin to disengage from care altogether — not because they don't want help, but because the structure meant to support them keeps falling apart.

What Veterans Are Entitled To

You are entitled to:

- A clearly assigned PACT team
- Proactive management of your care
- Reasonable continuity with your primary provider
- Same-day access for urgent or acute concerns
- Communication that respects your role as a full member of the team

When these things aren't happening, you're not asking for special treatment by speaking up — you're asking the VA to meet the minimum standards it has already committed to in writing.

Section 3 — How to Respond When PACT Fails You

When your PACT team fails to deliver timely, consistent, and coordinated care, you have more than just a complaint — you have a policy-backed case. The VA has codified the responsibilities of PACT providers in VHA Handbook 1101.10(2). That means when the system doesn't follow through, you don't need to argue your opinion — you can point to specific obligations the VA has failed to meet.

Step 1: Document the Breakdown

Start by writing down what happened, when it happened, and who was involved. Key items to track:

- Missed or canceled appointments
- Unexpected reassignment of your PCP or team members
- Delays in returning secure messages or phone calls
- Failures to provide same-day care
- Gaps in follow-up, like unreviewed test results or uncoordinated referrals

Note dates, names, and any communication attempts you made. These entries will form the foundation of your complaint.

Step 2: Reference the Handbook

Use **direct language from VHA Handbook 1101.10(2)** to strengthen your position. For example:

- *"According to Section 8(d)(6), my PACT team is required to ensure same-day access for urgent concerns, but I was not offered a same-day appointment or a call back."*
- *"Section 8(d)(8) requires that non-emergency care be directed first to my assigned provider. I've been seen by multiple random providers without explanation."*

This transforms your frustration into a policy-based grievance.

Step 3: Contact the Patient Advocate or Clinic Administrator

Submit a written complaint to the VA Patient Advocate or primary care clinic supervisor. Keep your tone respectful, but direct. Include:

- A brief summary of what happened
- How the situation violates PACT policy
- The specific section(s) of the handbook that were not followed
- What resolution you're requesting (e.g., assignment back to a prior provider, clarification of your current team, or improvement in access)

Request a written response and keep a copy of your submission.

Step 4: Use Secure Messaging and MyHealtheVet Notes

Send a secure message to your PACT team (and save a copy) summarizing your concern. Example:

> "I am requesting clarification of my assigned provider and care team. I have seen three different providers in my last four visits and have not been informed of any official change in assignment. This seems to violate the continuity of care required by VHA Handbook 1101.10(2), Sections 3 and 8. Please advise."

You can also write a note in MyHealtheVet after an appointment to document what occurred — this can later serve as useful evidence if the problem persists.

Step 5: Escalate if Needed

If no one responds or the problem continues, escalate the issue to:

- The primary care service chief or facility director
- The VISN-level Patient Advocate
- The Office of the Inspector General (OIG) if you believe the issue reflects systemic or willful noncompliance

Refer back to Chapters 7 and 8 of this guide for step-by-step escalation templates and strategies.

Section 4 — How to Request a New Provider Without Losing Access

Inconsistent care is frustrating, but not all breakdowns require a formal complaint. Sometimes the issue is simple: you've lost confidence in your provider, feel dismissed, or communication has broken down. In these cases, requesting a new provider may be the most effective path forward — but it's important to do it strategically so you don't lose access to care or disrupt continuity further.

Know That Reassignment Is Allowed

There is no policy that prevents you from asking for a new provider. However, VA facilities typically handle these requests carefully to ensure resources are balanced and continuity is preserved.

Your right to coordinated care — as outlined in VHA Handbook 1101.10(2) — includes being part of a care team that respects your values, preferences, and communication style. If that trust is broken, it's legitimate to ask for reassignment.

How to Request the Change Professionally

Make your request clear, respectful, and focused on care. Avoid personal attacks or emotional language. Instead, highlight your goal of maintaining continuity with a team that fits your needs. Example language:

> "*I appreciate the care I've received, but I believe a different provider may be a better fit for my communication needs and long-term care goals. I'm requesting reassignment within the same PACT team or to a provider with availability for ongoing continuity of care.*"

Put this in writing — either through a secure message, a MyHealtheVet request, or a letter to the clinic administrator. Keep a copy.

What to Expect After Your Request

Your facility may:

- Offer a meeting with the current provider or team to resolve concerns first
- Assign you to another provider within the same PACT (often the covering PCP)
- Place you on a waitlist if capacity is limited

If your request is denied or ignored, escalate using the tools from Chapter 4 — but in most cases, a respectfully written, care-focused request is honored without resistance.

If You're Pressured Not to Switch

Some Veterans are told things like:

- "*We don't allow provider changes unless there's a major issue.*"
- "*You'll have to wait months to see someone else.*"
- "*You should stick with this team to maintain continuity.*"

If you experience this, respond firmly but professionally:

> "*Continuity is important to me — that's why I'm requesting a provider who I feel I can build trust with. According to VHA Handbook 1101.10(2), the PACT model is built on patient-centered*

> *care and shared decision-making. I'm requesting reassignment in that spirit."*

Document your request and any response you receive. If necessary, submit a formal written complaint.

Section 5 — What to Do When the VA Changes Your Provider Without Notice

Few things are more disruptive than building a relationship with a primary care provider, only to find out they've been reassigned — often without warning, explanation, or input. These silent reassignments erode trust and directly violate the principles of continuity outlined in VHA Handbook 1101.10(2).

VHA Handbook 1101.10(2) does not allow the VA to reassign you casually or without explanation. While provider changes do happen (due to transfers, staffing changes, or performance issues), the PACT model requires continuity and transparency.

According to the Handbook:

- Continuity of care is essential to good outcomes, especially for chronic conditions.

- Veterans are entitled to a consistent, coordinated team, not a revolving door of providers.

- The team must respect and involve the Veteran in decisions, including provider assignment when possible.

If your provider is reassigned without notice or justification, this is a breach of the VA's own care model. Below is a step-by-step guide on how to respond to an unauthorized provider reassignment:

Step 1: Check Your Records

- Log into MyHealtheVet and confirm who is listed as your assigned provider.

- Look at your recent visit summaries or messages. Was the new provider introduced formally, or were you switched without discussion?

Step 2: Ask for Clarification

Send a secure message to the PACT team or call the clinic directly:

> "*Can you please confirm who my assigned primary care provider is? I was recently scheduled with a different provider without any explanation, and I'd like to understand whether I've been reassigned and why.*"

Step 3: Request Reinstatement or Formal Reassignment

If you want to return to your previous provider (and they're still available), submit a formal request:

> "*I was not informed of any official reassignment and would like to remain under the care of [previous provider], if possible. I value the continuity of that relationship, which aligns with the PACT model as outlined in VHA Handbook 1101.10(2).*"

If that provider is no longer available, request to be assigned to someone long-term — not temporarily.

Step 4: Escalate if Needed

If your inquiry is ignored or denied without proper explanation:

- Contact the Patient Advocate
- Submit a written complaint to the clinic administrator
- Reference VHA Handbook 1101.10(2), Sections 3 and 8 regarding continuity and reassignment transparency

Include any MyHealtheVet notes, secure messages, or scheduling history as evidence.

Keep Your Paper Trail

Just like with missed follow-up care or communication breakdowns, provider reassignments without notice should always be documented. Keep a detailed timeline of when you first noticed the change, any responses you received from VA staff, and any complaints or reassignment requests you submitted. A strong paper trail gives you power—and if you need to escalate further (as outlined in Chapter 4), it becomes the foundation of your case.

Section 6 — The Link Between PACT Failures and VA Medical Errors

When your PACT team doesn't follow through—whether it's failing to return messages, neglecting follow-up care, or bouncing you between providers—the consequences can go far beyond frustration. These breakdowns often serve as the root causes of serious medical errors. In fact, research within and outside the VA system has shown that fragmented care, poor communication, and lack of continuity are leading contributors to delayed diagnoses, medication mistakes, and preventable hospitalizations. The PACT model was specifically designed to prevent these outcomes by assigning each Veteran to a stable care team, supporting same-day access, and using tools like secure messaging and shared health records to ensure coordination across visits. But when PACT teams fail to uphold their responsibilities, the model collapses—and Veterans pay the price.

These failures can be subtle at first but build over time. A diabetic patient doesn't receive timely lab follow-up because no one on the team is clearly assigned to monitor it. A substitute provider adjusts a Veteran's medication without fully understanding their history, leading to dangerous side effects. A request for specialty care gets lost because no one responds to secure messages. In each of these cases, the harm wasn't caused by a single oversight, but by a pattern of inattention—a system that fails to do what it claims to do.

That's why documentation is so important. If you experience medical harm or serious disruption in care, the VA might try to treat it as an isolated incident. But with a clear paper trail—secure messages, appointment records, phone logs—you can show that the harm was the result of a systemic failure, not a random mistake. That distinction matters greatly, particularly if you're considering a formal complaint, an appeal, or even a tort claim under the Federal Tort Claims Act (FTCA). Even if you're not ready to escalate, having the evidence gives you power: it gives you credibility when you ask for change—and leverage when you demand accountability.

Section 7 — When to Report PACT Failures to Leadership or the OIG

Not every problem with a PACT team needs to be escalated. But when the same issues happen repeatedly—like ignored messages, unexpected provider reassignments, or long delays for urgent care—it's time to act. These aren't just inconveniences; they're violations of your rights under VHA Handbook 1101.10(2). And when internal complaints go nowhere, it's appropriate to take your concerns higher.

Begin by submitting a clear, written complaint to your facility's Primary Care Service Chief or Medical Center Director. Outline what went wrong, when it happened, and who was involved. More importantly, cite the sections of the handbook that were violated—especially those related to continuity of care, same-day access, and team communication. Attach a timeline or log of events, including secure messages and appointment history, to show this isn't an isolated incident.

If local leadership fails to respond or resolve the problem, your next step is to contact your VISN-level Patient Advocate. Each VISN has designated officials responsible for addressing unresolved patient concerns. Don't hesitate to ask for their contact information through the medical center's main line or website.

For serious or systemic failures—especially if patient safety is involved—you can file a report directly with the VA Office of the Inspector General (OIG) using their public hotline. In your report, focus on policy violations, patterns of negligence, or instances where VA staff knowingly failed to meet documented responsibilities. Upload relevant complaint records, screenshots, and responses to strengthen your submission.

In extreme cases, especially when health or benefits are at risk, contacting your Congressional representative is another option. A congressional inquiry can prompt a review from senior VA officials and create accountability where internal channels have failed.

Whatever level of escalation you choose, your documentation is your leverage. A well-organized complaint supported by VA policy and your personal record of what occurred shifts the burden of accountability where it belongs—onto the system that promised to care for you.

The Patient Aligned Care Team (PACT) model was designed to make VA primary care more responsive, more coordinated, and more Veteran-centered. On paper, it offers a level of access and continuity many private systems still struggle to match. But as you've now seen, those promises are only real when the VA follows its own policies — and when Veterans know what those policies actually require.

Whether it's same-day access, communication with your assigned provider, or transparency in how your care is managed, VHA Handbook 1101.10(2) is not just an internal guide. It's a powerful tool you can use to protect your health, assert your rights, and hold your care team accountable.

When your provider is reassigned without notice, when your messages go unanswered, or when your urgent concerns are dismissed — you now have the language, the policy, and the process to respond.

Remember: This system is supposed to work for you. And when it doesn't, your job is not to accept less — your job is to make the system face the standards it wrote for itself.

PART VI —Final Thoughts and References

> *"The VA — Giving Veterans a second chance to die for their country since 1930."*
> *(Veteran humor, but not far from reality.)*

It's a harsh joke—but it exists for a reason. It speaks to the frustration, disillusionment, and betrayal that many Veterans feel after trusting a system that doesn't always honor its promises.

This part of the book steps back to reflect—not just on what's broken, but on how you reclaim your power, sharpen your voice, and build something stronger than what failed you. You've learned how to read the system, how to challenge it, and how to lead others through it with clarity and conviction. Now it's time to think about what comes next—and how you'll carry that strength forward.

These final chapters are about recognition, solidarity, and action. About understanding that you are not alone—and that the path forward doesn't require perfection, only persistence.

Let's close the book with strength, purpose, and a reminder: what you've endured doesn't define you. What you choose to do next does.

Chapter 18: Becoming a Veteran Advocate for Others

There comes a point in every Veteran's VA journey when frustration gives way to clarity. At first, you're just trying to make the system work. You're calling for appointments, chasing down referrals, trying to get your records fixed, and wondering if anyone at the VA is actually listening. For most of us, that stage lasts longer than it should.

But if you stay in the fight long enough, something shifts. You stop feeling helpless. You begin to see patterns. You notice when staff bend or break the rules. You learn the difference between what should happen and what actually does. And then, one day, another Veteran turns to you and says, "How did you do it?"

That's when you realize: you're not just a patient anymore. You're becoming an advocate.

Advocacy Starts Small

> Most advocacy doesn't begin with a mission statement. It starts with a hallway conversation. A friend asking for help filing a complaint. A fellow Veteran unsure how to request their records. Someone who didn't even know they could challenge what was written in their chart.
>
> You don't have to know everything. Just showing someone where to look can be enough. Share the name of a directive. Help them write their first secure message. Tell them what a patient advocate is supposed to do—and what to do if they don't. These moments matter. They build trust, confidence, and courage in people who may have been dismissed or gaslit by the system for years.
>
> Sometimes, the most powerful thing you can do is listen. Just saying, "*You're not crazy. That shouldn't have happened*," can open a door that's been shut for too long.

Teaching What You've Learned

Once you've fought your own battles, you begin to realize how few Veterans understand their rights or how the system is supposed to work. You can change that—one person at a time.

Teach them how to:

- Access and read their full VA medical record, including nursing intake notes
- Spot misleading entries or gaps in documentation
- File amendment requests under VHA Directive 1605.01
- Use VHA Directive 1003.04 to hold Patient Advocates accountable
- Identify where breakdowns in communication or care coordination are likely to occur

You don't need to have all the answers. Just pointing someone in the right direction, sharing what worked for you, and being willing to walk a few steps with them is often enough.

Guarding Your Boundaries

Helping others is rewarding—but it can also be draining. If you've been through the fight yourself, you know how much energy it takes. As you begin to help others, protect your time and emotional bandwidth. You can guide someone without taking on their whole case. You can teach without carrying.

Set clear expectations. Say, *"I'll help you write your first complaint, but you need to send it."* Or, *"I'll show you how to find the directive, but I can't read your whole record."*

Veteran-to-Veteran advocacy is most effective when it's empowering, not enabling. Help others find their voice, not just borrow yours.

Building Veteran-to-Veteran Networks

One of the most important lessons I learned is this: when we advocate together, we stop being isolated cases. We become proof of a pattern. When multiple Veterans begin to notice the same failures—the same bad policies, the same misused documentation templates, the same non-responsive advocates—something shifts. It stops feeling like your fault, and starts looking like what it is: a systemic failure.

That's why small, local Veteran networks matter. They can form anywhere: in a town hall, in a waiting room, on a Facebook group. Veterans who start comparing notes soon discover they're not alone—and that they're stronger together.

These informal groups don't need to be big. A few people willing to share their stories, compare documentation, or coordinate complaints can make a real impact. At my local clinic, the Bay Pines Town Hall became the starting point for something bigger—a community of Veterans finally realizing they weren't imagining the problem. And that they could do something about it.

Helping Others Helps You Heal

There's a reason this chapter belongs here, at the end of the book. Advocacy isn't just a tool for fixing the system—it's a way to reclaim yourself.

For me, helping others gave meaning to what I went through. It turned frustration into clarity. Pain into purpose. And silence into strategy. When you help someone else, you're no longer stuck inside your own story. You see that what you endured can spare someone else. You learn that your voice has power.

You may not get recognition. The system may still try to ignore you. But that doesn't erase the difference you make when you help another Veteran find their footing. You've walked the hard road. You know the barriers. That makes you the best kind of guide.

You Were Never Just a Patient

You were always more than what the VA saw on paper. More than a checklist, more than a score, more than what was left out of your chart.

You were never just a patient. You were a witness. And now, you're an advocate.

That matters.

Because the next Veteran who comes through the doors is going to need someone who knows the way.

Chapter 19: Working Toward System-Level Change

It starts with one case. One Veteran denied care they clearly earned. One record filled with misleading entries. One advocate who refuses to get involved. But as you begin helping others, you start to see what the VA often wants you to miss: it's not just a series of unfortunate events. It's a pattern.

That's when the real shift happens. You move beyond correcting individual errors. You start asking bigger questions: Why do these failures keep happening? Who is responsible for fixing them? And what would it take to ensure no other Veteran goes through the same thing?

That shift marks the beginning of system-level advocacy—a form of engagement that doesn't just push back against personal injustice, but works to change the conditions that allowed it in the first place.

Why Systems Matter

Most of the problems described in this book aren't random. They stem from how the VA organizes its care, manages its people, and responds to accountability. Whether it's boilerplate denials from the Privacy Office or Patient Advocates who simply forward complaints without action, these issues reflect deeper flaws in leadership culture, training protocols, and performance metrics.

If a nurse can falsely document your record and face no consequence—if a provider can ignore a diagnosis because it doesn't fit their narrative—if a facility can violate its own directives without external scrutiny—then the system itself is enabling harm. That's what has to change.

Connecting Cases to Patterns

To create change, you have to document it. That means:

- Collecting similar experiences across multiple Veterans
- Comparing language in denials, notes, and intake records
- Citing violations of specific VA policies and directives
- Tracking whether repeated issues were addressed or ignored

When you can show that a breakdown isn't isolated—but repeated, widespread, and policy-violating—you're no longer presenting a complaint. You're presenting evidence of a system failure.

This is where your advocacy turns a corner. You stop asking for exceptions. You start demanding reform.

Escalating with Purpose

Every failed resolution at the local level is an invitation to escalate. And you have more tools than you might think:

- VISN (Veterans Integrated Service Network) leadership offices
- The VA Office of Inspector General (OIG)
- Congressional caseworkers and field reps
- Veteran Service Organizations (VSOs) with legislative reach

Each of these channels has strengths and limitations. Use them strategically. Keep your records clean, your tone professional, and your claims well-sourced. Provide timelines, quotes, and clear references to directives or law. If you can link the same violations across multiple Veterans, your case becomes much harder to ignore.

Building Coalitions, Not Just Cases

The VA counts on Veterans staying isolated—on each of us fighting our own private battle, with no time or energy to look around. When Veterans begin connecting, comparing, and coordinating, the whole equation changes.

Coalition-building doesn't require a national organization. It can start with a few Veterans who:

- Share similar problems at the same facility
- Write complaints together to show consistent patterns
- Appear at town halls to give public voice to shared concerns
- Elevate each other's stories when contacting Congress

Over time, these coalitions can become catalysts. They give weight to what might otherwise be dismissed as a lone Veteran's opinion. They push leadership to confront what they'd rather keep hidden. They amplify not just complaints, but calls for accountability.

Don't Wait for Permission

> The VA won't ask you to be part of the solution. In fact, if you're vocal enough, they may treat you as the problem. But that doesn't change the truth: no one understands the VA's failures better than the Veterans who've lived through them. And no one is better positioned to fix it than those who care enough to try.

Change never starts at the top. It begins with people who are willing to speak the truth, demand better, and refuse to give up.

The system isn't going to fix itself. But that's not the end of the story.

It's the start of your next mission.

Chapter 20: Finding Strength in Shared Veteran Experience

The most dangerous lie the system tells you is that you're alone. Of course, it is not said that way. It sounds more like this:

> *"Your case is an exception."*
>
> *"I think that you misunderstood what happened."*
>
> *"I understand you are not happy with the outcome…"*

You may be fighting a system that says that your story isn't believable. Or use your frustration against you to make you to be just bitter, angry, or ungrateful.

But the truth is something else entirely. The truth is that thousands of Veterans have been through what you've been through—or something close to it. And many of them are still quietly struggling, still trying to make sense of why the system failed them, and still wondering if it was somehow their fault.

It wasn't.

You didn't imagine the dismissals, the delays, or the denials. You didn't imagine being blamed for your own injuries, being told to "just move on," or being treated like a number instead of a human being. And you're not imagining the toll it's taken on your mind, your body, your family, or your faith.

You are not alone.

Real Strength Isn't Silence

> Too many Veterans were taught that strength means staying quiet. Pushing through. Not complaining. Taking the hit and moving on.
>
> But strength isn't silence. Real strength is knowing when to speak up. When to call out what's wrong. When to admit you need help—and when to help someone else who does.
>
> Real strength is continuing to show up, even after the system has failed you. It's choosing to use your experience not just as a scar, but as a source of guidance for others. It's not about being perfect. It's about being honest.

The Power of Shared Experience

When you tell your story, you make it easier for someone else to tell theirs. You create space. You build trust. You remind people that they're not crazy for being hurt by something that should have helped them.

This book has shared strategies, policies, and step-by-step guidance. But what matters just as much is the spirit behind it: the decision to no longer suffer in silence, and the belief that by sharing what you've learned, you can spare others the same pain.

Veterans supporting Veterans isn't a program. It's a lifeline.

The Strength of Staying in the Fight

You may not win every battle. The VA may not admit its mistakes. Even when you do win, it may take time. Some of my wins took almost a year. But every time you show up—for yourself, for someone else, or for the principle of accountability—you chip away at the silence that protects dysfunction.

You force the system to see you. And sometimes, that's the first step to making it change.

Whether you're writing a complaint, mentoring a fellow Veteran, showing up at a town hall, or simply sharing what you've learned—you are doing the work. You are forcing the system to correct itself.

Closing Words

If there's one thing I want you to take away from this book, it's that you're not alone — and you never were.

You're not the only one who's been ignored, blamed, or sent in circles. You're not the only one who's had to fight for what should have been standard. And you're not the only one who's asked: *Is it just me?*

It's not just you.

You're part of a growing number of Veterans who are beginning to see the pattern, speak up about it, and support each other through it. Some are just starting out. Some have been fighting for years. But together, we are forming something stronger — a shared understanding that the system can and must do better.

You may not have all the answers yet. But you know enough to make a difference — for yourself and for someone else.

So stay alert. Get connected. And get organized.

Because when we support each other, the system has to pay attention.

And that's what real strength looks like.

Appendices

Appendix A: Key VA Directives, Laws, and Regulations Referenced

This appendix provides a quick-reference list of foundational laws, directives, and policies that Veterans can cite in complaints, appeals, and accountability efforts. Each entry includes a brief summary and practical application.

---

5 U.S. Code § 552a - Records maintained on individuals (The Privacy Act)

- **What it is:**
  This federal law governs how federal agencies — including the Department of Veterans Affairs — must manage, maintain, and disclose personal records. It guarantees individuals the right to:
    - Access their own records held by federal agencies,
    - Request amendments to incorrect or incomplete information,
    - Receive a formal response within specific timelines,
    - File a statement of disagreement if an amendment is denied, and
    - Ensure that all future disclosures include a notation about disputed information.

- **Why It Matters:**
  For Veterans, this law is the legal backbone of your right to fix false or misleading entries in your VA medical record. If VA refuses to amend inaccurate documentation — even after clear evidence — this statute gives you the right to escalate the issue and force a formal review. It also ensures your side of the story is recorded and disclosed alongside any disputed information. This law empowers you to protect your record and assert your credibility when accessing care or applying for benefits.

- **Where to find:**
  https://www.law.cornell.edu/uscode/text/5/552a

38 U.S. Code § 7309A — Patient Advocacy Program

- **What it is**:
  This federal statute formally established the Office of Patient Advocacy within the Department of Veterans Affairs. It defines the legal authority, responsibilities, and operational expectations for all Patient Advocates within the VA health care system. The law requires Patient Advocates to:
  - **Advocate on behalf of Veterans** regarding their VA health care experiences,
  - **Resolve complaints** that cannot be addressed at the point of service,
  - **Track, report, and analyze complaint data**, and
  - **Understand and educate Veterans** on their health care rights, responsibilities, and available appeals.

- **Why it matters**:
  This law gives Veterans the legal right to expect true advocacy from VA Patient Advocates — not just passive complaint logging. When advocates dismiss, delay, or deflect concerns, this statute provides the foundation for demanding accountability. It also mandates that advocates receive training, document complaints in a national tracking system, and bring serious or recurring issues to VA leadership. Citing this law reinforces that advocacy inside the VA isn't optional — it's a legal obligation.

- **Where to find:**
  https://www.law.cornell.edu/uscode/text/38/7309A

38 C.F.R. § 0.603 — Principles of Veteran Customer Experience

- **What it is**:
  This federal regulation outlines how the Department of Veterans Affairs is required to deliver services — including health care — based on three measurable principles of customer experience: **Ease**, **Effectiveness**, and **Emotion**. These are not just internal goals; they are **codified standards** that apply to **every interaction** a Veteran or caregiver has with the VA. The regulation also ties customer experience directly to VA's core values ("I CARE") and mandates the use of customer feedback data to drive improvement.

- **Why it matters**:
  This law gives Veterans the right to expect accessible, competent, and respectful service. It provides a legal foundation for filing complaints when care is delayed, communication is poor, or staff are dismissive. By citing § 0.603, Veterans can hold the VA accountable for violating federally defined service standards — not just being "unhelpful." It elevates a poor experience into a regulatory compliance issue, making it a powerful tool when advocating for corrective action or service recovery.

- **Where to find:**
  https://www.ecfr.gov/current/title-38/chapter-I/part-0/subpart-A/section-0.603

38 C.F.R. § 1.579 — Amendment of Records

- **What It Is:**
  This VA regulation outlines the **official process for requesting amendments** to personal records maintained by the Department of Veterans Affairs. It implements provisions of the Privacy Act (5 U.S.C. § 552a) specific to the VA and mandates that:
    - Veterans can request correction of inaccurate, incomplete, untimely, or irrelevant records,
    - VA must acknowledge the request within **10 business days**,
    - VA must respond with a final decision within **30 business days**, or explain any delay,
    - Veterans may **appeal a denial** and submit a **statement of disagreement**,
    - VA must **mark disputed records** and include the Veteran's statement with any future disclosures.

- **Why It Matters:**
  This regulation is central to protecting your **reputation, benefits eligibility, and medical credibility**. If a VA record contains false, misleading, or incomplete information — especially in clinical notes — this rule provides the legal basis for **demanding correction**. It also ensures your version of the events is added to your official record if VA refuses to amend it. For any Veteran trying to fix damaging entries, challenge unfair denials, or prepare for appeals, this regulation is a critical tool in the fight for accountability.

- **Where to find:**
  https://www.ecfr.gov/current/title-38/chapter-I/part-1/subject-group-ECFR457b46c49efc094/section-1.579

38 C.F.R. § 17.38 Medical benefits Package

- **What It Is:**
This regulation defines the official scope of health care services that enrolled Veterans are entitled to receive under the VA's "medical benefits package." It includes both basic and preventive care, such as:
    - Inpatient and outpatient medical, surgical, and mental health care
    - Prescription medications, prosthetics, and rehabilitative devices
    - Emergency and home health services
    - Maternity and newborn care (with limits)
    - Counseling for family members
    - Completion of certain forms based on clinical evaluation

- **Why It Matters:**
This regulation is the foundation for what VA is required to provide to eligible Veterans. When a Veteran is told "we don't do that here," this rule can be used to verify whether the service is actually included — and to challenge improper denials. It also supports complaints or escalation efforts when medically necessary services are delayed or denied. Importantly, it confirms that form completion (e.g., SSDI, FMLA, private disability) is part of the care VA is authorized to deliver — a critical fact often misunderstood by staff. This regulation empowers Veterans to demand medically appropriate care, not just accept whatever is offered.

- **Where to find:**
https://www.ecfr.gov/current/title-38/chapter-I/part-17/subject-group-ECFRf01c7718f2a7e24/section-17.38

VHA Directive 1003 — Veteran Patient Experience

- **What it is**:
  VHA Directive 1003 (2020) establishes national policy and responsibilities for ensuring a consistent, high-quality patient experience across all VA medical facilities. It defines the principles of Veteran Patient Experience based on Ease, Effectiveness, and Emotion and mandates a structured, system-wide approach involving every VA employee. The directive incorporates service recovery, patient advocacy, employee training, and continuous improvement practices to drive cultural transformation and operational accountability.

- **Why it matters**:
  This directive matters because it creates enforceable expectations for how Veterans are treated throughout their care journey in the VA system. It mandates that every interaction—from scheduling appointments to resolving complaints—must reflect the VA's core values and build trust. By defining patient experience as a measurable performance priority and linking it to leadership accountability and training, the directive gives Veterans and caregivers a powerful tool to advocate for respectful, responsive, and transparent service. It also reinforces that all VA staff—not just advocates—are responsible for ensuring a positive Veteran experience and prompt service recovery.

- **Where to find:**
  https://www.va.gov/vhapublications/ViewPublication.asp?pub_ID=8789
  If that link stops working in the future, Try searches like 'site:va.gov VHA Directive 1003' or 'Patient Experience policy site:va.gov' to quickly find the official version.

VHA Directive 1003.04 — Patient Advocacy

- **What it is**:
  This directive establishes the official policy and procedures for the VA Patient Advocacy Program across all VA health care facilities. It requires Patient Advocates to:
    - Proactively advocate on behalf of Veterans and resolve concerns,
    - Serve as a point of contact for Veterans' rights and complaints,
    - Document all issues in the national tracking system (PACT),
    - Escalate unresolved concerns to leadership, and
    - Educate staff and Veterans on how to use the program.

  It defines who is responsible at every level, from front-line advocates to facility directors and VISN leadership, and sets expectations for timeliness, resolution, and follow-up.

- **Why it matters**:
  This directive is essential because it confirms that VA Patient Advocates are not just passive messengers — they are required to act. It gives Veterans the right to expect active, structured, and accountable assistance when problems arise. If an advocate dismisses your complaint, delays action, or says they "don't advocate," this directive proves otherwise. It provides the basis for holding the advocacy program — and facility leadership — accountable when VA services fail to meet legal or policy standards. It is one of the most powerful tools in this guide for turning passive complaints into meaningful action.

- **Where to find:**
  https://www.va.gov/vhapublications/ViewPublication.asp?pub_ID=11548
  If that link stops working in the future, Try searches like 'site:va.gov VHA Directive 1003.04' or 'Patient Advocacy site:va.gov' to quickly find the official version.

Appendix A

VHA Directive 1110.02 — Social Work Professional Practice

- **What it is**:
  This directive defines the national policy and scope of VA Social Work Services, outlining the roles, responsibilities, and functions of social workers across the Veterans Health Administration. It mandates that social workers:
    - Advocate for and assist Veterans and caregivers in accessing services,
    - Provide case management, crisis intervention, and discharge planning,
    - Facilitate access to community resources and benefits,
    - Support vulnerable populations, including homeless Veterans, those with serious mental illness, and survivors of military sexual trauma (MST),
    - Serve as part of the **treatment team** to promote whole health and patient-centered care.

- **Why it matters**:
  This directive confirms that VA social workers have a formal duty to advocate for Veterans — especially those facing barriers to care. Whether you are being denied MST-related services, need coordinated home or community care, or require support during a crisis, this directive proves that social work is not optional or auxiliary — it is integrated and mandated. When other parts of the system fail, this policy gives Veterans the right to request social work involvement to help navigate benefits, programs, and appeals. It's a vital tool when the system becomes too complex or unresponsive.

- **Where to find:**
  https://www.va.gov/vhapublications/ViewPublication.asp?pub_ID=11912
  If that link stops working in the future, Try searches like 'site:va.gov VHA Directive 1110.02' or 'Social Work site:va.gov' to quickly find the official version.

Appendix A

VHA Directive 1134(2) — Completion of DBQs and Forms by VA Providers

- **What it is:**
  This directive requires VA health care providers to complete both VA and non-VA medical forms and provide medical statements when requested by a Veteran, provided it's within their scope of practice and clinical knowledge. It covers forms such as:
  - Disability Benefits Questionnaires (DBQs),
  - Family Medical Leave Act (FMLA) forms,
  - Social Security Disability forms,
  - Aid & Attendance applications,
  - Work status and return-to-duty forms.

- **Why it matters:**
  This directive provides clear, enforceable rights for Veterans who are often told, "We don't fill out forms." It ensures that form refusal, delay, or evasion by VA providers is not permitted under national policy. For Veterans applying for SSDI, housing assistance, VA benefits, or other support, this rule is essential for accessing timely and complete documentation. Citing this directive can compel VA staff to honor requests and prevent Veterans from falling through administrative cracks.

- **Where to find:**
  https://www.va.gov/vhapublications/ViewPublication.asp?pub_ID=4300
  If that link stops working in the future, Try searches like 'site:va.gov VHA Directive 1134' or 'Completion of forms site:va.gov' to quickly find the official version.

VHA Directive 1445 — Whole Health System

- **What it is**:
  This directive establishes the VA's national policy for implementing the Whole Health System of Care, which shifts the focus of care from "What's the matter with you?" to "What matters to you?" It requires all VA medical centers to:
    - Offer Veterans personal health planning centered around life goals and values,
    - Provide access to well-being services (e.g., yoga, tai chi, nutrition, coaching),
    - Integrate Whole Health into clinical care delivery, using team-based support and complementary services,
    - Train staff and Veterans on Whole Health principles, tools, and resources.

  The system includes three core elements: the Pathway (exploration of purpose), Well-Being Programs, and Whole Health Clinical Care.

- **Why it matters**:
  This directive is a powerful tool for Veterans who feel dismissed, rushed, or reduced to diagnoses. It guarantees your right to care that respects your priorities, values, and long-term goals — not just your symptoms. If your providers ignore requests for integrative care, dismiss your well-being priorities, or bypass shared decision-making, you can cite this directive to demand participation in the Whole Health model. It also reinforces your right to request services like health coaching, mind-body therapies, and personalized care planning as part of your treatment — not just optional extras.

- **Where to find:**
  https://www.va.gov/vhapublications/ViewPublication.asp?pub_ID=11498

  If that link stops working in the future, Try searches like 'site:va.gov VHA Directive 1445' or 'Whole Health System site:va.gov' to quickly find the official version.

VHA Directive 1605.01 — Privacy and Release of Information

- **What it is:**
  This directive outlines the VA's national policy on privacy, confidentiality, and the release of Veterans' personal health and benefit information. It implements the requirements of the Privacy Act, HIPAA, and other federal laws, ensuring that:
    - Veterans have the right to access their own records,
    - Records are only released with appropriate authorization or legal authority,
    - Staff are trained and held accountable for protecting privacy,
    - Veterans can request amendments to their records under specific procedures,
    - The VA must notify individuals in case of privacy breaches. It also defines the roles and responsibilities of Privacy Officers at all VA facilities.

- **Why it matters:**
  This directive reinforces that your medical and personal information belongs to you — not to VA staff. It guarantees your right to access your records, to challenge inaccurate documentation, and to control how and when your information is shared. When VA personnel delay your records request, refuse to explain what's in your file, or fail to protect your private data, this directive gives you a clear legal foundation to demand accountability. It's especially important when dealing with records amendments, My HealtheVet downloads, third-party form requests, or breaches of confidentiality.

- **Where to find:**
  https://www.va.gov/vhapublications/ViewPublication.asp?pub_ID=11388
  If that link stops working in the future, Try searches like 'site:va.gov VHA Directive 1605.01' or 'Privacy and Release of Information site:va.gov' to quickly find the official version.

VHA Handbook 1101.10(2) — Patient Aligned Care Team (PACT) Handbook

- **What it is:**
  This handbook defines the Patient Aligned Care Team (PACT) model, which is VA's official system for delivering primary care. It requires every enrolled Veteran to be assigned to a care team consisting of:
    - A primary care provider,
    - A registered nurse care manager,
    - A clinical associate (e.g., LPN or medical assistant),
    - An administrative clerk.

  The PACT model is designed to provide patient-centered, proactive, coordinated care that emphasizes continuity, communication, same-day access, and preventive services. It also encourages shared decision-making and care tailored to the Veteran's goals and needs.

- **Why it matters:**
  This handbook is crucial because it outlines what every Veteran should expect from their VA primary care team. If you're experiencing fragmented care, poor communication, or lack of follow-through, this document gives you a solid basis to demand improvement. It shows that care coordination, follow-up, and access to your provider's team are not luxuries — they are VA-mandated standards. This is especially useful when filing complaints, requesting reassignment, or escalating unresolved issues with your care team.

- **Where to find:**
  https://www.va.gov/vhapublications/ViewPublication.asp?pub_ID=2977

  If that link stops working in the future, Try searches like 'site:va.gov VHA Directive 1101.10(2)' or 'Patient Aligned Care Team site:va.gov' to quickly find the official version.

VA Handbook 6300.4 — Procedures for Processing Requests for Records Subject to the Privacy Act

- **What it is:**
  This handbook lays out the official step-by-step procedures the VA must follow when a Veteran requests to:
    - Access records about themselves,
    - Amend or correct information in those records,
    - Receive disclosures or explanations regarding their privacy rights,
    - Appeal a denial of access or amendment.

  It implements the federal Privacy Act of 1974 and ensures VA compliance in handling personally identifiable information (PII), including rules for disclosure, corrections, appeal rights, and criminal penalties for mishandling data.

- **Why it matters**:
  This handbook gives Veterans a procedural roadmap for correcting false or harmful information in their VA records. It's essential for Veterans who have experienced inaccurate documentation—whether in medical, benefits, or administrative files. The handbook spells out what the VA is legally required to do, including deadlines, appeal options, and the role of Privacy Officers. If your request to fix a record is delayed, denied, or ignored, you can point directly to the procedures in this handbook to hold the VA accountable and assert your rights.

- **Where to find:**
  https://www.va.gov/vapubs/viewPublication.asp?Pub_ID=701&FType=2

  If that link stops working in the future, Try searches like 'site:va.gov VA Directive 6300.4' or 'Processing Requests for Records Subject to the Privacy Act site:va.gov' to quickly find the official version.

Appendix B: VA Terms Every Veteran Should Know

ADLs (Activities of Daily Living)
Basic self-care tasks like bathing, dressing, toileting, transferring, and eating. These are often documented in evaluations for SMC, caregiver eligibility, or long-term care.

CBOC (Community-Based Outpatient Clinic)
Smaller local clinics operated by the VA, usually focused on primary care, mental health, and basic lab services. These do not offer emergency or specialty care.

Community Care
Medical services provided by private-sector doctors but paid for by the VA, used when VA cannot provide timely care or needed services in-house. Must be approved through a consult and authorization process.

Congressional Inquiry
A formal request submitted through your U.S. Senator or Representative's office to investigate or resolve issues with the VA. VA facilities are required to respond promptly and formally to these inquiries.

DBQ (Disability Benefits Questionnaire)
A standardized medical form used by VA (or private) providers to evaluate a Veteran's condition for disability claims. VA providers are required to complete these when appropriate under VHA Directive 1134.

MyHealtheVet
The VA's online portal for managing appointments, prescriptions, secure messaging, and medical records. *Critical for documentation and tracking care.*

No Wrong Door Policy
A VHA principle that staff should never send a Veteran away without helping — even if it's "not their department." Referenced in patient experience policy.

OIG (Office of Inspector General)
An independent body within the VA that investigates fraud, abuse, and systemic failure. *Use when other escalation routes fail.*

PACT (Patient Aligned Care Team)
Your VA primary care team, typically including a provider, nurse case manager, LPN, and clerical support. They coordinate your care and referrals. *Problems here often cause delays elsewhere.*

Patient Advocate
An official role created by Congress to help resolve barriers to care inside the VA health care system. Their duties include investigating complaints, coordinating with staff, and reporting systemic failures. Governed by 38 U.S.C. § 7309A and VHA Directive 1003.04.

Priority Group (PG)
A tiered system used by the VA to determine your level of access and cost of care. Lower numbers (e.g., PG 1) mean higher priority and fewer copays.

Process Improvement
A leadership-driven mandate to identify and correct recurring system failures within the VA. Used in conjunction with data from Patient Advocates and complaints.

Process Improvement Team
The internal team responsible for reviewing systemic failures and implementing corrective actions based on data and patient complaints.

Secure Messaging (MyHealtheVet)
An encrypted messaging system within the VA portal that allows Veterans to communicate with their care teams. *One of the most important tools for documentation.*

Service Chief
The clinical or administrative leader of a service line (e.g., Chief of Primary Care). A key escalation point before going to facility or VISN leadership.

Service Line
A division or department within a VA facility (e.g., Primary Care Service Line, Mental Health Service Line). Complaints are often routed here — sometimes improperly — without resolution.

Service Recovery
A required VA process for resolving care breakdowns (e.g., lost referrals, appointment delays). Every VA facility must have a Service Recovery Program under VHA Directive 1003.

The Braden Scale
A standardized nursing tool used to assess risk for pressure ulcers. Used during nursing intake to assess skin risk. Often misused as a proxy for independence level, leading to misleading entries about Veteran function.

VA Medical Center (VAMC)
A full-service VA hospital offering primary care, specialty care, surgery, and inpatient services. Often serves as the hub for smaller outpatient clinics.

VBA (Veterans Benefits Administration)
Handles disability claims, compensation, pensions, education, housing, and insurance — *this is where your claim decisions are made*.

Veteran Experience Officer
An official assigned to oversee the Veteran Patient Experience at each VA Medical Center. Often misperceived as a purely symbolic role but has policy oversight duties under VHA Directive 1003.

VHA (Veterans Health Administration)
The branch of the VA responsible for providing health care services. It operates hospitals, clinics, community care, and manages patient records — *this is where you receive your care*.

VISN (Veterans Integrated Service Network)
A regional management layer of the VA health care system that oversees multiple VA Medical Centers. Each VISN has its own leadership and is responsible for performance, budgeting, and oversight — *a key escalation point when local facilities fail*.

Appendix C: Complaint Templates and Examples

Every Veteran case is different, but strong complaints tend to follow similar structures. This appendix gives you working templates and real examples you can adapt to your situation. These are based on what has actually worked for Veterans who pushed their concerns to VA leadership, VISN, the Office of the Inspector General (OIG), and Congressional offices.

Each example below is structured with clarity, professionalism, and a clear connection to VA policy or federal law. Use these as a foundation — just swap in your specific facts, timelines, and policy citations as needed.

Template 1 — Complaint to Patient Advocate Supervisor or Medical Center Director

Subject: Urgent: Complaint Not Addressed in Accordance with VHA Directive 1003.04

Dear [Patient Advocate Supervisor/Medical Center Director Name],

I am writing to formally request action on a complaint I submitted on [date] regarding [brief summary of issue]. Despite raising this concern through the Patient Advocate Office, I have yet to receive a response that aligns with the duties outlined in VHA Directive 1003.04.

Specifically, the directive states that Patient Advocates must coordinate resolution in partnership with service lines and provide timely, actionable updates (Paragraphs 2(l)(2) and 2(l)(5)). As of today, these responsibilities appear unmet.

I am requesting written clarification on how this matter is being resolved, and by whom.

Thank you for your attention,

[Full Name]
[Last Four of SSN]
[VA Facility & PACT Team]
[Phone / Email]

Template 2 — Congressional Inquiry Request

Subject: Request for Assistance with Ongoing VA Health Care Issue

Dear [Congressional Staff Member or Office of Representative ____],

I am a Veteran enrolled in VA health care at [VA Medical Center]. I am requesting your office's help in initiating a Congressional inquiry regarding unresolved access to care and noncompliance with VA policy.

Issue: Despite multiple attempts to resolve [brief issue summary], I have been unable to obtain [needed care, service, response]. My concerns were submitted to the Patient Advocate Office, but I have not received a meaningful resolution.

Policy Violated: VHA Directive 1003.04 requires Patient Advocates to coordinate resolution, ensure timely updates, and assist with care access. These steps have not occurred.

I respectfully request that your office ask for a formal response from VA leadership and review whether proper procedures were followed. Supporting documentation is provided in Appendix A.

Thank you for your advocacy.

[Full Name]
[Last Four of SSN]
[Phone / Email]
[VA Facility]

Template 3 — OIG Complaint (Formal)

Subject: Formal Complaint: Systemic Noncompliance with VHA Directive 1003.04

To Whom It May Concern,

I am submitting this complaint to formally report a pattern of systemic failure at [VA Facility], specifically involving the Patient Advocacy Program's lack of compliance with VHA Directive 1003.04.

Despite repeated attempts to engage with the Patient Advocate Office to resolve [brief issue], my concerns have not been acted on. The required coordination with service lines did not occur, nor was I provided timely or complete updates as outlined in Paragraphs 2(l)(2) and 2(l)(5) of the directive.

This failure has contributed to a delay in care with potentially serious health consequences. All internal channels have been exhausted, and documentation of my efforts is included in the appendices.

I respectfully request the Office of Inspector General investigate the handling of this matter and determine whether corrective action is warranted.

[Full Name]
[Last Four of SSN]
[VA Facility & PACT Team]
[Phone / Email]
[Date of Most Recent Complaint Attempt]

The best way to learn how to write effective complaints is to see how others have done it — and what actually gets attention at each level of escalation. The following examples walk through real-world scenarios that begin with a common problem and show how that issue can be systematically elevated through the VA chain of command, to VISN leadership, to a congressional office, and finally to the Office of Inspector General (OIG). These aren't just stories — they are models you can follow. Each example shows how to start at the lowest appropriate level, use policy-based language to make your case, and adapt your escalation strategy based on urgency, risk, and inaction. Use these examples as a blueprint, and remember: your documentation and persistence make all the difference.

Example 1 — Missed Referral to Cardiology Escalation Steps

Issue: Veteran was referred by their PCP for cardiology, but the appointment was never scheduled. Months pass with no communication.

- **Step 1:** Veteran asks Patient Advocate to investigate.
- **Step 2:** Advocate says scheduling is not their responsibility.
- **Step 3:** Veteran escalates to the Patient Advocate Supervisor, then the Patient Experience Officer with policy references to VHA Directive 1003.04 on coordination of care.
- **Step 4:** Veteran contacts the Medical Center Director.
- **Step 5:** No results. Veteran writes to VISN leadership requesting intervention.
- **Step 6:** Veteran's congressional office submits an inquiry citing care delay.
- **Step 7:** Veteran files a complaint with the OIG documenting failure to act despite internal escalation.

Complaint to Patient Advocate Supervisor:

Subject: Missed Cardiology Referral – Request for Resolution

Dear [Supervisor Name],

On [Date], my VA Primary Care Provider referred me to Cardiology for further evaluation. As of today, that appointment has not been scheduled, and I've received no communication from scheduling or the specialty clinic. I previously contacted the Patient Advocate Office, but was told this issue does not fall under their responsibility.

This delay poses a serious risk to my health and reflects a breakdown in care coordination. Per VHA Directive 1003.04, Patient Advocates are required to coordinate with service lines to help resolve complaints and access issues. I am requesting that this matter be addressed promptly and documented accordingly.

Sincerely, [Veteran Name]

Complaint to Patient Experience Officer:

Subject: Unresolved Cardiology Referral – Patient Safety Concern

Dear [PXO Name],

I am writing to escalate an unresolved issue involving my cardiology referral from [Date]. Despite repeated efforts, including contact with the Patient Advocate Supervisor, I have not received a scheduled appointment.

Given the ongoing delay and potential health risk, I request your immediate review and assistance. VHA Directive 1003.04 outlines your responsibility to oversee complaint resolution efforts that impact Veteran experience and care access.

Sincerely, [Veteran Name]

Letter to Medical Center Director:

Subject: Formal Complaint – Missed Cardiology Referral and Noncompliance with VHA Policy

Dear Director [Name],

I am submitting a formal complaint regarding an unfulfilled referral to Cardiology. Despite proper clinical referral from my PCP, the specialty appointment has not been scheduled. My previous complaints through Patient Advocacy and the Patient Experience Office have gone unresolved.

I respectfully request intervention under VHA Directive 1003.04, which outlines coordination responsibilities for complaint resolution. This failure jeopardizes my health and violates VA's duty of care.

Sincerely, [Veteran Name]

Letter to VISN Leadership:

Subject: Escalation Request – Medical Center Failure to Schedule Cardiology Referral

Dear VISN 08 Director,

I am requesting intervention from your office regarding a breakdown in care coordination. Despite being referred to Cardiology months ago and submitting complaints to the Patient Advocate Supervisor, Patient Experience Officer, and Medical Center Director, no appointment has been scheduled.

This unresolved issue poses a significant health risk. I ask that your office review this matter under VHA policy and ensure corrective action.

Sincerely, [Veteran Name]

Letter to Congressional Office:

Subject: Request for Congressional Assistance – Unfulfilled VA Cardiology Referral

Dear [Congressional Staffer],

I am requesting your assistance with an ongoing VA health care issue. I was referred to Cardiology by my VA doctor on [Date], but the appointment has never been scheduled. Despite escalating through the Patient Advocate chain and Medical Center leadership, no resolution has been provided.

I believe this delay poses a risk to my health and violates VA policies for timely care coordination. I respectfully request your office submit a formal inquiry to help secure timely medical care.

Sincerely, [Veteran Name]

OIG Complaint:

Subject: Failure to Schedule Specialty Care – Risk to Veteran Health

Dear Office of Inspector General,

I am submitting a formal complaint regarding VA's failure to fulfill a Cardiology referral made by my Primary Care Provider on [Date]. I have documented communications with the Patient Advocate, Patient Experience Officer, Medical Center Director, VISN office, and congressional office, yet no appointment has been scheduled.

This represents a pattern of neglect that endangers my health and violates VHA Directive 1003.04 regarding care coordination and complaint resolution. I request an investigation into this failure and systemic scheduling breakdowns.

Sincerely, [Veteran Name]

Example 2 — False Information in Medical Record Escalation Steps

Issue: A nurse inserted false information into the medical record that contradicts test results and physician documentation.

- **Step 1:** Veteran requests correction via the Patient Advocate.
- **Step 2:** Advocate defers to clinical staff. No action taken.
- **Step 3:** Veteran escalates to the Patient Advocate Supervisor, then to the Patient Experience Officer citing HIPAA and VHA Directive 1605.01.
- **Step 4:** Veteran sends formal complaint to the Medical Center Director.
- **Step 5:** With no response, Veteran contacts VISN leadership.
- **Step 6:** Congressional office submits an inquiry requesting policy compliance.
- **Step 7:** Veteran sends OIG a complaint citing compromised data integrity and clinical risk.

Complaint to Patient Advocate Supervisor:

Subject: Request to Correct Inaccurate Information in Medical Record

Dear [Supervisor Name],

I am writing to request correction of false information added to my VA medical record by [nurse's name] on [date]. The note claims [brief summary of false content], which contradicts both my diagnostic test results and documentation from my treating physician on [date].

I previously submitted a request for correction to the Patient Advocate Office, but no action has been taken. Under VHA Directive 1605.01 and HIPAA, I have the right to request correction of protected health information that is inaccurate or misleading.

Please ensure this matter is reviewed and that I am notified of the resolution process. I am prepared to provide supporting records.

Sincerely,
[Veteran Name]

Complaint to Patient Experience Officer:

Subject: Follow-Up – Inaccurate Medical Record and Failure to Act

Dear [PXO Name],

I'm writing to follow up on my previous request to correct inaccurate information in my medical record, submitted to the Patient Advocate Supervisor. No resolution has been provided, and the false entry remains in my file.

VHA Directive 1605.01 provides Veterans the right to request amendment of incorrect information. Additionally, failure to act undermines the accuracy and trustworthiness of VA records. I respectfully request your direct involvement.

Sincerely,
[Veteran Name]

Letter to Medical Center Director:

Subject: Formal Complaint – Inaccurate Medical Record Entry and Noncompliance with VHA 1605.01

Dear Director [Name],

I am submitting a formal complaint concerning a false entry in my VA medical record created by [nurse's name] on [date]. The content conflicts with clinical findings and my physician's notes, yet no correction has been made despite multiple requests.

This issue violates the standards outlined in VHA Directive 1605.01, Section 13, regarding the right of the individual to request amendment of protected health information. I request immediate review, correction of the inaccurate entry, and assurance this issue is addressed appropriately.

Sincerely,
[Veteran Name]

Letter to VISN Leadership:

Subject: Escalation – Medical Center Failure to Address Inaccurate Medical Record Entry

Dear VISN 08 Director,

I am escalating a concern involving the refusal of [VA Medical Center] to address an inaccurate and harmful medical record entry made by a nurse on [date]. Despite submitting formal requests through the Patient Advocate Supervisor, Patient Experience Officer, and Medical Center Director, the false entry remains uncorrected.

VHA Directive 1605.01 gives Veterans the right to request corrections. I request your assistance in ensuring the facility meets its obligations and protects the integrity of medical records.

Sincerely,
[Veteran Name]

Letter to Congressional Office:

Subject: Request for Assistance – Inaccurate Medical Record and Lack of VA Accountability

Dear [Congressional Staffer],

I'm seeking your help regarding an unresolved issue with the [VA Medical Center] involving false information in my VA medical record. I've gone through the appropriate channels — including the Patient Advocate Supervisor, Patient Experience Officer, and Medical Center Director — but no corrective action has been taken.

VHA Directive 1605.01 grants Veterans the right to request correction of false or misleading information. I believe my case deserves further review and accountability, and respectfully request your office initiate a congressional inquiry.

Sincerely,
[Veteran Name]

OIG Complaint:

Subject: Inaccurate VA Medical Record Entry and Refusal to Comply with HIPAA and VHA Policy

Dear Office of Inspector General,

I am reporting an unresolved issue involving a false entry in my VA medical record at [VA Medical Center] by a nurse on [date], which contradicts objective clinical evidence. My formal requests for correction, submitted to the Patient Advocate, PXO, Medical Center Director, and VISN, have been ignored or denied without adequate explanation.

This refusal violates HIPAA and VHA Directive 1605.01 and represents a risk to clinical decision-making and patient safety. I request an investigation into the systemic failure to uphold medical record accuracy and patient rights.

Sincerely,
[Veteran Name]

Example 3 — Doctor Refuses to Fill SSDI Form Escalation Steps

Issue: Veteran's doctor refuses to complete SSDI paperwork, claiming it violates VA policy.

- **Step 1:** Veteran submits complaint to Patient Advocate.
- **Step 2:** Advocate says providers can decline at their discretion.
- **Step 3:** Veteran escalates to the Supervisor, then to the Patient Experience Officer referencing VHA Directive 1134.
- **Step 4:** Veteran files a complaint to the Medical Center Director.
- **Step 5:** After no meaningful response, the Veteran escalates to VISN leadership.
- **Step 6:** Congressional office submits inquiry to obtain required documentation.
- **Step 7:** Veteran files complaint with OIG to review systemic denial of required assistance.

Complaint to Patient Advocate Supervisor:

Subject: Provider Refusal to Complete SSDI Forms – Request for Clarification and Assistance

Dear [Supervisor Name],

I recently asked my VA provider, [Doctor's Name], to complete SSDI documentation needed by my attorney for my disability case. I was told this is against VA policy because it might involve a future court appearance. This directly contradicts what I understand to be VA policy under VHA Directive 1134, which requires providers to complete medically appropriate forms that support a Veteran's disability claims when within their scope of practice.

I request your assistance in confirming the policy and ensuring that I receive the support I am entitled to. Please review this matter and advise me on how the VA intends to resolve it.

Sincerely,
[Veteran Name]

Complaint to Patient Experience Officer:

Subject: Escalation – Improper Denial of SSDI Form Completion by VA Provider

Dear [PXO Name],

I am escalating a concern regarding my VA provider's refusal to complete SSDI disability paperwork that my attorney submitted. The provider stated this is against VA policy. However, VHA Directive 1134 clearly outlines the responsibilities of VA health care professionals to complete forms that assist in supporting a Veteran's disability applications.

This issue directly affects my financial stability and right to access federal benefits. I request your immediate assistance in reviewing this refusal and facilitating an appropriate resolution.

Sincerely,
[Veteran Name]

Letter to Medical Center Director:

Subject: Formal Complaint – Refusal to Complete SSDI Form in Violation of VHA Directive 1134

Dear Director [Name],

I am submitting a formal complaint regarding my VA provider's refusal to complete Social Security Disability paperwork. The explanation provided was that this might require the provider to appear in court, which was cited as a reason to decline assistance.

According to VHA Directive 1134, providers are required to complete appropriate documentation to assist Veterans in obtaining federal, state, or local benefits, including SSDI. This refusal violates VA policy and denies me necessary support in a time of need.

I respectfully request immediate review and resolution of this matter.

Sincerely,
[Veteran Name]

Letter to VISN Leadership:

Subject: Escalation – VA Provider's Refusal to Complete Disability Form in Violation of VHA Policy

Dear VISN 08 Director,

I am writing to escalate a policy violation at [VA Medical Center] involving my provider's refusal to complete SSDI documentation. My previous efforts to resolve this through the Patient Advocate, PXO, and Medical Center Director have not led to any correction or assistance.

VHA Directive 1134 explicitly requires that VA providers complete documentation to support Veteran disability claims when appropriate. The facility's failure to enforce this directive has placed my disability application at risk.

I request your intervention to ensure the Medical Center follows established VA policy and supports Veterans appropriately.

Sincerely,
[Veteran Name]

Letter to Congressional Office:

Subject: Request for Congressional Assistance – VA Refusal to Complete SSDI Forms

Dear [Congressional Staffer],

I need your assistance with a VA issue involving the refusal of my provider at [VA Medical Center] to complete SSDI paperwork for my disability claim. Despite referencing VHA Directive 1134, which supports Veterans receiving assistance with benefit-related forms, my request has been repeatedly denied without justification.

This denial is affecting my ability to obtain needed financial support. I respectfully request that your office initiate a congressional inquiry to ensure that VA staff fulfill their duties and support Veterans seeking disability benefits.

Sincerely,
[Veteran Name]

OIG Complaint:

Subject: Systemic Noncompliance – VA Refusal to Complete SSDI Disability Documentation

Dear Office of Inspector General,

I am submitting a formal complaint involving the refusal of VA medical staff at [VA Medical Center] to complete my SSDI disability forms, in direct contradiction to VHA Directive 1134. My provider stated this violates VA policy due to possible legal exposure, but the directive clearly requires such documentation to be completed when within the scope of clinical practice.

I have exhausted internal channels, including the Patient Advocate, PXO, Medical Center Director, VISN, and Congressional Office. This appears to be a systemic failure to follow VA policy and fulfill VA's responsibilities to its disabled Veteran population.

I respectfully request investigation into this ongoing issue.

Sincerely,
[Veteran Name]

Appendix D: Complaint Strategy Quick Reference Table

Quick Reference Table: Choosing the Right Complaint Strategy

Complaint Target	Primary Purpose	Tone to Use	What to Include
Patient Advocate Supervisor	Address poor handling of a complaint by front-line PAs	Firm but cooperative	Cite VHA Directive 1003.04; describe unresolved issue; request corrective action
Patient Experience Officer	Address systemic or repeated breakdowns in Veteran care	Professional and focused	Highlight patterns; cite VHA Directives 1003 & 1003.04; request oversight or intervention
Medical Center Director	Demand accountability from facility leadership	Direct and fact-driven	Summarize failed steps; reference policy violations; state harm or ongoing risk
VISN Leadership	Escalate above local facility for regional intervention	Formal and concise	Outline unresolved issues; cite relevant directives; include attachments or appendix
Congressional Office	External oversight for serious or unaddressed concerns	Respectful and clear	Provide plain-language summary; show failed attempts to resolve; attach policy-based evidence

Appendix E: Logging VA Contacts and Building Your Paper Trail

Log Template You Can Start Using Today

Date	Action Taken	VA Response	Policy Involved	Next Step
07 Apr 25	Secure msg to PCP re: lost neurology consult	No response by 17 Apr 25	VHA Dir 1003 (Timeliness)	Follow-up msg, CC Patient Advocate
18 Apr 25 09:20	Call to Patient Advocate Office – spoke w/ Mr. James	Stated "consults are backlog-related" but offered no ETA	38 U.S.C. § 7309A, VHA Dir 1003.04	Email summary to Mr. James; request written plan
30 Apr 25	Email to Service Chief (Neuro) labelled Escalation	Awaiting reply	VHA Dir 1232(2) (Referral processing)	Escalate to Med Ctr Director if no reply by 10 May

Why a Log Changes the Power Dynamic

Without a Log	With a Log
"I called a few times and no one got back to me."	"On **April 8** at **14:15**, I phoned Neurology; **Ms. Flores** stated the consult 'was still pending,' contradicting CPRS notes printed the same day."
Staff deny delays or blame other departments.	You cite exact dates, names, and relevant policy each step of the way.
Leadership can minimize the issue as an isolated case.	Your timeline reveals a pattern—evidence of systemic failure, not a one-off glitch.

Digital vs. Paper

- **Digital spreadsheet** (Excel, Google Sheets) makes sorting and filtering easy, and you can attach files or cloud links.

- **Notebook** works if you're more comfortable handwriting; just photograph or scan pages so you can email them later.

- **MyHealtheVet Download**: You can download your secure-message history to attach as exhibits—another built-in audit trail.

How Often to Update

- **Immediately** after any call or clinic visit—while details are fresh.

- **Weekly** review: highlight entries older than 14 days with no response; these become your next follow-ups.

- **Before every escalation**: skim the log, copy the most relevant line items into your email so leadership sees the time stamps.

Turning the Log Into Leverage

When you escalate, paste a concise excerpt:

"Attached timeline shows four unanswered contacts between 07 Apr 25 and 30 Apr 25. This pattern violates the timeliness requirements in VHA Directive 1003. I request immediate service-recovery action and a written plan of correction."

Leadership now confronts hard data, not anecdote. Ignoring that data risks their own performance metrics—and they know it.

Appendix F: Commonly Cited USC, CFR, VHA Directives and Handbooks

5 U.S. Code § 552a - Records maintained on individuals (The Privacy Act)

(d) (2) permit the individual to request amendment of a record pertaining to him

(d) (2)(B)(i) make any correction of any portion thereof which the individual believes is not accurate, relevant, timely, or complete

(d)(2)(B)(ii) inform the individual of its refusal to amend the record in accordance with his request, the reason for the refusal, the procedures established by the agency for the individual to request a review of that refusal by the head of the agency or an officer designated by the head of the agency, and the name and business address of that official

(d)(3) permit the individual who disagrees with the refusal of the agency to amend his record to request a review of such refusal. And if, after his review, the reviewing official also refuses to amend the record in accordance with the request, permit the individual to file with the agency a concise statement setting forth the reasons for his disagreement with the refusal of the agency, and notify the individual of the provisions for judicial review of the reviewing official's determination under subsection (g)(1)(A) of this section.

38 U.S. Code § 7309A - Office of Patient Advocacy

(c)(2)(A) In carrying out the Patient Advocacy Program of the Department, the Director shall ensure that patient advocates of the Department advocate on behalf of Veterans with respect to health care received and sought by Veterans under the laws administered by the Secretary.

(d)(1) The responsibilities of each patient advocate at a medical facility of the Department are the following: To resolve complaints by Veterans with respect to health care furnished under the laws administered by the Secretary that cannot be resolved at the point of service or at a higher level easily accessible to the Veteran.

(d)(3) The responsibilities of each patient advocate at a medical facility of the Department are the following: To express to Veterans their rights and responsibilities as patients in receiving such health care.

(d)(8) The responsibilities of each patient advocate at a medical facility of the Department are the following: To ensure that any significant complaint by a Veteran with respect to such health care is brought to the attention of appropriate staff of the Department to trigger an assessment of whether there needs to be a further analysis of the problem at the facility-wide level.

(d)(11) The responsibilities of each patient advocate at a medical facility of the Department are the following: To understand all laws, directives, and other rules with respect to the rights and responsibilities of Veterans in receiving such health care, including the appeals processes available to Veterans.

38 CFR - chapter 1 – Part 0 – Subpart A — Core Values, Characteristics, and Customer Experience Principles of the Department

§ 0.601 Core Values.

VA employees should adopt this motto and these Core Values in their day-to-day operations.

(a) **Integrity**. VA employees will act with high moral principle, adhere to the highest professional standards, and maintain the trust and confidence of all with whom they engage.

(b) **Commitment**. VA employees will work diligently to serve Veterans and other beneficiaries, be driven by an earnest belief in VA's mission, and fulfill their individual responsibilities and organizational responsibilities.

(c) **Advocacy**. VA employees will be truly Veteran-centric by identifying, fully considering, and appropriately advancing the interests of Veterans and other beneficiaries.

(d) **Respect**. VA employees will treat all those they serve and with whom they work with dignity and respect, and they will show respect to earn it.

(e) **Excellence**. VA employees will strive for the highest quality and continuous improvement, and be thoughtful and decisive in leadership, accountable for their actions, willing to admit mistakes, and rigorous in correcting them.

§ 0.602 Core Characteristics.

The Core Characteristics define what VA stands for and what VA strives to be as an organization.

(a) **Trustworthy**. VA earns the trust of those it serves, every day, through the actions of its employees. They provide care, benefits, and services with compassion, dependability, effectiveness, and transparency.

(b) **Accessible**. VA engages and welcomes Veterans and other beneficiaries, facilitating their use of the entire array of its services. Each interaction will be positive and productive.

(c) **Quality**. VA provides the highest standard of care and services to Veterans and beneficiaries while managing the cost of its programs and being efficient stewards of all resources entrusted to it by the American people. VA is a model of unrivalled excellence due to employees who are empowered, trusted by their leaders, and respected for their competence and dedication.

(d) **Innovative**. VA prizes curiosity and initiative, encourages creative contributions from all employees, seeks continuous improvement, and adapts to remain at the forefront in knowledge, proficiency, and capability to deliver the highest standard of care and services to all of the people it serves.

(e) **Agile**. VA anticipates and adapts quickly to current challenges and new requirements by continuously assessing the environment in which it operates and devising solutions to better serve Veterans, other beneficiaries, and Service members.

(f) **Integrated**. VA links care and services across the Department; other federal, state, and local agencies; partners; and Veterans Services Organizations to provide useful and understandable programs to Veterans and other beneficiaries. VA's relationship with the Department of Defense is unique, and VA will nurture it for the benefit of Veterans and Service members.

§ 0.603 Customer Experience principles.

Customer experience is the product of interactions between an organization and a customer over the duration of their relationship. VA measures these interactions through Ease, Effectiveness, and Emotion, all of which impact the overall trust the customer has in the organization.

(a) **Ease.** VA will make access to VA care, benefits, and memorial services smooth and easy.

(b) **Effectiveness.** VA will deliver care, benefits, and memorial services to the customer's satisfaction.

(c) **Emotion.** VA will deliver care, benefits, and memorial services in a manner that makes customers feel honored and valued in their interactions with VA. VA will use customer experience data and insights in strategy development and decision making to ensure that the voice of Veterans, servicemembers, their families, caregivers, and survivors inform how VA delivers care, benefits, and memorial services.

38 C.F.R. § 1.579 — Amendment of Records

(a) Any individual may request amendment of any VA record pertaining to him or her. The VA will promptly either:
  1. Correct any part thereof which the individual believes is not accurate, relevant, timely or complete; or
  2. Inform the individual of the VA refusal to amend the record in accordance with his or her request, the reason for the refusal, the procedures by which the individual may request a review of that refusal by the Secretary or designee, and the name and address of such official.

(c) Any individual who disagrees with the VA refusal to amend his or her record may request a review of such refusal. If, after review, the Secretary or designee also refuses to amend the record in accordance with the request the individual will be advised of the right to file with the VA a concise statement setting forth the reasons for his or her disagreement with the VA refusal and also advise of the provisions for judicial review of the reviewing official's determination.

(d) In any disclosure, containing information about which the individual has filed a statement of disagreement, the VA will clearly note any part of the record which is disputed and provide copies of the statement (and, if appropriate, copies of a concise statement of the VA's reasons for not making the amendments requested) to persons or other agencies to whom the disputed record has been disclosed.

38 § 17.38 Medical benefits package

(a)(1)(xv) Completion of forms (e.g., Family Medical Leave forms, life insurance applications, Department of Education forms for loan repayment exemptions based on disability, non-VA disability program forms) by healthcare professionals based on an examination or knowledge of the Veteran's condition, but not including the completion of forms for examinations if a third party customarily will pay health care practitioners for the examination but will not pay VA.

(a)(2) Preventive care

   vi. Prevention of musculoskeletal deformity or other gradually developing disabilities of a metabolic or degenerative nature.
   vii. Genetic counseling concerning inheritance of genetically determined diseases.
   viii. Routine vision testing and eye-care services.
   ix. Periodic reexamination of members of high-risk groups for selected diseases and for functional decline of sensory organs, and the services to treat these diseases and functional declines.
   x. Chiropractic services.

VHA Directive 1003 — Veteran Patient Experience

Section 4. POLICY

It is VHA policy that all levels of the organization understand and are accountable for how their roles and responsibilities affect the Veteran Patient Experience and ensure every employee adheres to the Core Values, Characteristics, and Veteran Patient Experience Principles of VA, to provide the best experience possible to Veterans, Servicemembers, their families, caregivers, and survivors.

Section 5. RESPONSIBILITIES

(j) VA Medical Facility Personnel. All VA medical facility personnel are responsible for:

    (1) Demonstrating commitment to VA Core Values, Characteristics, and Customer Experience Principles of the VA according to employee performance plan standards.

    (2) Complying with this directive and Veteran Patient Experience-related VA policies.

Section 6. SERVICE RECOVERY

(b) Effective Service Recovery programs contain the following components:

    (1) A process that is user-friendly and allows easy access for Veterans to voice complaints.

    (2) A personalized Service Recovery experience that involves the Veteran in the decision or resolution.

(c) Principles. Principles of Service Recovery include:

    (1) Focusing on achieving fairness and true Veteran satisfaction.

    (2) Anticipating and correcting problems before they occur.

    (3) Acknowledging mistakes without placing blame or making excuses.

    (4) Apologizing for not meeting service expectations.

    (5) Taking corrective actions in a timely manner.

    (6) Ensuring appropriate follow-up and feedback to the Veteran

VHA Directive 1003.04 — Patient Advocacy

Section 1. POLICY

It is VHA policy that patient advocacy, as a fundamental value in VHA's culture, considers the needs, preferences, priorities and values of Veterans in a proactive and convenient manner.

Section 2. RESPONSIBILITIES

- (i) VA medical facility Service Chiefs are responsible for:
  - (2) Providing oversight of complaints assigned to the service line in PATS and ensuring timely resolution based on designated timeframes and quality documentation that supports complaint closure.
  - (3) Ensuring timely entry and resolution of complaints by Service Level Advocate(s) (SLA).
- (j) The VA medical facility Patient Advocate Supervisor is responsible for:
  - (4) Providing JIT training and support to VA medical facility employees in understanding: (a) The responsibility each employee has, to advocate on behalf of Veterans.
  - (6) Ensuring that Patient Advocates enter and close patient complaints in PATS based on designated timeframes and provide documentation that addresses the complaint.
- (l) The VA medical facility Patient Advocate is responsible for:
  - (2) Coordinating resolution for complaints that cannot be resolved at the point of service or require assistance from multiple service lines.
  - (3) Notifying the VA medical facility Patient Advocate Supervisor when very difficult or challenging complaints have been identified and more support is needed.
  - (4) Providing guidance and support to SLAs in their efforts to address complaints in PATS, within their service line, by the designated timeframe.

VHA Directive 1110.02 — Social Work Professional Practice

Section 2. RESPONSIBILITIES

(p) VA medical facility social worker is responsible for (1) Providing social work services to include:
 (f) Advance care planning and goals of care conversations.
 (g) Resource referral and community services coordination.
 (i) Community care and community resource linkage.
 (j) Interdisciplinary collaboration, coordination, and consultation.
 (m) Patient, family, caregiver, and survivor education.
 (n) Client advocacy.

VHA Directive 1134(2) — Provision of Medical Statements and Completion of Forms by VA Health Care Providers

Section 4. POLICY

Except when specifically prohibited, it is VHA policy that providers, when requested, must assist patients in completion of VA and non-VA medical forms and provide medical statements with respect to the patient's medical condition and functionality.

Section 5. RESPONSIBILITIES

(d) The VA medical facility Director is responsible for:
  (1) Establishing processes and procedures addressing the following:
    (a) VA health care providers are responsible for completing VA medical forms. Examples of VA medical forms completed upon patient or beneficiary request include, but are not limited to:
    (c) Completion of DBQs to Support VA Benefits Claims. A "no wrong door" philosophy must be adopted to accommodate Veterans bringing a VA DBQ form to a VA medical facility for completion.
    (d) Completion of Non-VA Medical Forms. Patients may ask VA health care providers, including primary care and specialty providers, to complete non-VA forms that require a medical professional's assistance or medical opinion.
      (1) Examples of non-VA forms include, but are not limited to:
        a. Family Medical Leave Act forms
        b. Life insurance application forms
        c. Non-VA disability retirement forms
        d. Return to work/work status forms
        e. Medical clearance forms
        f. State and federal workers' compensation forms
        g. Permits (e.g. state driver's license, handicap parking forms)
        h. Medical necessity or accommodation forms (e.g., for equipment or supplies, transit, utilities, etc.)

    i. Capacity evaluation forms (e.g., functional, mental health, etc.)
    j. Social Security Administration (SSA) examination forms
    k. Death certificates
    m. Attorneys' forms regarding patient medical status or functional assessment
 (e) The facility Chief of Staff and Associate Director for Patient Care Services are responsible for:
  (1) Ensuring that VA providers understand their responsibility for providing medical statements and completing VA and non-VA forms in accordance with this directive.
  (3) Developing alternative strategies for situations when completion of a form extends beyond the scope of a VA provider or when completion of a form would disrupt the therapeutic relationship
 (f) VA providers are responsible for:
  (1) Completing VA and non-VA forms and medical statements received from or on behalf of patients with respect to a patient's medical condition and functionality, to the best of their ability based on their scope and clinical expertise. When completion of the form extends beyond the scope of the provider, the provider should assist by consulting with a specialty care expert as appropriate, reviewing evidence in the VA electronic medical record (including text documents, test results and vital measurements) pertinent to the condition and function that provides important information needed to complete medical forms and statements.
  (3) Seeking further guidance and assistance from the designated facility MS&F POC, Risk Manager, Privacy Officer, or other facility representatives, when necessary, to address questions or issues that may arise while completing medical statements or VA and non-VA forms.

VHA Directive 1445 — Whole Health System

Section 1. POLICY

It is VHA policy that the Whole Health System (WHS) is integrated at all VA medical facilities so that Veterans have access to a model of care that empowers and equips them to take charge of their health and well-being and to live their lives to the fullest.

Section 2. RESPONSIBILITIES

- (h) The VA medical facility Director is responsible for:
    - (1) Ensuring overall VA medical facility compliance with the directive and appropriate corrective action is taken if non-compliance is identified.
    - (2) Ensuring resources, such as adequate staffing and personnel, are available for implementation of minimum WHS requirements at the VA medical facility.
- (n) The VA medical facility Health and Wellness Coach is responsible for:
    - (1) Supporting Veterans in mobilizing internal strengths and external resources to develop strategies for making sustainable, healthy lifestyle behavior changes and more effectively managing chronic disease.
    - (2) Working in close collaboration with interdisciplinary clinical and non-clinical staff and teams throughout the VA medical facility on a Veteran-centered process to facilitate and empower Veterans to develop and achieve self-determined goals related to health and well-being.
- (o) The VA medical facility Whole Health Partner is responsible for:
    - (1) Informing Veterans of available Whole Health services and recruiting Veterans to participate in Whole Health initiatives at the VA medical facility relevant to their Mission, Aspiration and Purpose (MAP) as they develop an individualized Personal Health Plan (PHP).
    - (2) Connecting Veterans to VA medical facility and community Whole Health resources.

VHA Handbook 1101.10(2) — Patient Aligned Care Team (PACT) Handbook

Section 6. PACT PRINCIPLES: PACT principles establish the foundation for high-quality primary care for Veterans and apply to all PACTs.

a. **Patient-centered Care.** Patient-centered care starts with the Veteran. Patient-centered care is personalized, proactive, and patient-driven health care. Patient-centered care focuses on discovering the Veteran's vision of living life fully and his or her goals for health. The PACT, including the Veteran and personal support persons, come together as partners to create the Veteran's plan for health. The team helps Veterans acquire the skills and resources they need to engage in self-care and self-management and provides Veterans with ongoing support and coaching needed to succeed in making and sustaining changes in their health.

b. **Team-Based Care.** Team-based care embraces the strong practice of teamwork among members dedicated to achieving the common goal of excellent comprehensive primary care for Veterans. The synergistic efforts of an effective team surpass the ability of any single individual to meet the health care needs of a panel of patients.

c. **Continuous Improvement.** PACT staff employs continuous improvement strategies and active learning to improve the team's function, increase efficiency, encourage standardization, improve health outcomes and optimize the quality of care they deliver.

d. **Data Driven Care.** Quality of care is based on the highest level of evidence available at the time, which may include data, expert opinion, consensus, and professionally accepted standards for the practice of care.

e. **Population Health and Prevention.** Population health refers to the "health outcomes of a group of individuals, including the distribution of such outcomes within the group". It is an approach designed to improve the health of an entire population of patients, and can also be applied to the subset of patients managed by a health care team, or to the patients cared for by a clinic or facility.

f. **Access and Timeliness.** Access and timeliness are essential components of high quality customer service and support VHA's goals to provide prompt and appropriate treatment for Veterans' health concerns. PACT staff works as a team to provide the right care at the right time in the right place by the right person.

g. **Comprehensiveness.** Comprehensiveness in primary care ensures that patients are offered all necessary and appropriate health care and are provided care in a manner consistent with the patient's (or surrogate's) treatment preferences and wishes.

h. **Care Coordination.** Care coordination by the PACT facilitates integration of health care services and navigation through complex health care systems. It involves working across care settings and accessing health care providers and other services, such as community programs to help patients receive the care they need and want without unnecessary duplication of services or avoidable inconvenience.

i. **Continuity of Care.** PACT staff establishes a caring longitudinal relationship with Veterans and personal support persons that persists beyond a single episode of care. Continuity of care means that one team is the point of contact for coordinating their patients' current and future VA health care.

Section 8. PACT OPERATIONS MANAGEMENT PROCESSES

d. Access Management

(1) Excellent access is a cornerstone of patient-centered care. Excellent access means PACT staff is available to provide appropriate clinical advice or care using appropriate modalities of health care delivery at the time patients want and need the advice or care.

(2) Every VHA site that provides primary care implements accepted access management principles and processes to ensure that Veterans receive care in a timely manner.

(3) All PACT staff share responsibility for creating and maintaining access for in-person, face-to-face encounters, group visits, telehealth, secure messaging and telephone encounters for the designated panel of patients.

(6) All PCPs and RNs must ensure they have same-day access (unless it is too late in the day as determined by the individual facility) for face-to-face encounters, telephone encounters and, when required by VHA guidance or policy, other types of encounters.

(8) Processes for managing patients' requests for non-emergency care and same-day access must implement the principle of continuity of care by preferentially directing requests for nonemergency care according to the following descending hierarchy of care providers:
  (a) The patient's assigned PCP and other assigned PACT staff;
  (b) The designated covering PCP and covering PACT staff;
  (c) Any PCP and any PACT staff; and
  (d) Next day appointment (if acceptable to the patient) with the patient's assigned or designated covering PCP and other PACT staff.

e. Care Management
  (2) Care management processes must be established that are sufficient to ensure that appropriate PACT staff:
    (a) Offers and provides appropriate care management services to patients assigned to the PACT.
    (b) Assesses factors impacting patients' health status, and works with the patient and personal support persons to manage care in a way that relieves constraints or barriers to desired health status.
    (c) Provides patients and personal support persons with health education and coaching, and engages them in developing strategies for managing their full range of health conditions.
    (d) Collaborates with appropriate PACT members to develop and implement personal health plans for individual patients and for cohorts of patients.

f. Care Coordination
  (1) Care coordination facilitates integration of health care services and navigation through complex health care systems. It involves working across care settings, accessing health care providers and other services such as community programs, to help patients receive the care they need and want without unnecessary duplication of services or avoidable inconvenience. Care coordination involves open communication among health care providers, legally permissible exchange of health care information, and logistical integration of health care encounters.

(2) Care coordination processes must be sufficient to ensure PACT staff, typically the RNCM or Clinical Associate, coordinates care for patients assigned to the PACT when patients are:
 (a) Admitted to hospital, Emergency Department (ED), or Community Living Center (CLC).
 (b) Discharged from hospital, ED, or CLC.
 (c) Re-assigned to or from another PACT.
 (d) Receiving care from provider(s) of specialty care.
 (e) Receiving care from several health care providers, including VA providers, VA-contract providers, or providers unaffiliated with VA (e.g., dual care).
 (f) Undergoing complex or high risk surgical or interventional procedures.
(3) Care coordination processes must ensure:
 (a) There is no lapse in care for the patient.
 (b) Relevant information is communicated to involved providers.
 (c) PACT staff knows about transitions of assigned patients between care settings and are involved when needed to facilitate safe, effective, and patient-centered transitions.
 (d) Health record information is made accessible to involved providers in a timely manner.
 (e) Clinically recommended care is integrated to avoid duplication, poor timing, or missed care opportunities.

VA Handbook 6300.4 — Procedures for Processing Requests for Records Subject to the Privacy Act

Section 3. PROCEDURES FOR HANDLING REQUESTS FOR ACCESS TO OR AMENDMENT OF RECORDS

- e. Processing requests for correction or amendment of records.
  - (1) An individual may request amendment of a record pertaining to him or her contained in a specific VA system of records by mailing or delivering the request to the office concerned. It must state the nature of the information in the record the individual believes to be inaccurate, irrelevant, untimely, or incomplete; why the record should be changed; and the amendment desired.
  - (2) Not later than business 10 days after the date of a request to amend a record, the VA official concerned will acknowledge in writing such receipt. If a determination for correction or amendment has not been made, the acknowledgement will inform the individual of when to expect information regarding the action taken on the request. VA will complete a review of the request to amend or correct a record within 30 business days of the date of receipt.
  - (3) Where VA agrees with the individual's request to amend his or her record(s), the requirements of 5 U.S.C. 552a(d) will be followed. The record(s) will be corrected promptly and the individual will be advised promptly of the correction.
  - (5) If it is determined not to grant all or any portion of the request to amend a record, the VA official will promptly notify the individual in writing. The individual will be advised of his or her right to file a concise statement of reasons for disagreeing with the refusal to amend. The VA notice will **specify the reason(s) for denying the request, identify the VA regulations or statutes upon which the denial is based**, and advise that the denial may be appealed in writing to the General Counsel.

(9) If the adverse determination is sustained by the General Counsel or Deputy General Counsel, the individual will also be advised promptly of his or her right to file a concise statement of reasons for disagreeing with the refusal to amend. The statement may contain information that the individual believes should be substituted.

(10) When an individual files a statement disagreeing with VA's decision not to amend a record, the record will be clearly annotated so that the fact that the record is disputed is apparent to anyone who may subsequently access, use, or disclose it. When the disputed record is disclosed to persons or other agencies, the fact of the dispute will be clearly noted. Copies of the statement of disagreement will be provided, and, when appropriate, copies of a concise statement of VA's reasons for not making the amendment(s) requested will also be provided.

Appendix G: How to File a Record Amendment

What the Law Guarantees You

Under **5 USC § 552a(d)(2)**, any individual may request the amendment of a federal record pertaining to them that they believe is:

- Inaccurate
- Irrelevant
- Untimely
- Incomplete

VA medical records fall under this law because they are part of a federal system of records. That means you can legally challenge any entry that distorts the truth — even if it's just poorly worded or paints the wrong picture.

The VA is then required to:

1. Acknowledge your request within 10 business days
2. Complete a review and provide a written response within 30 business days
3. If denied, inform you of your right to submit a written Statement of Disagreement
4. Include your disagreement in any future disclosures of the disputed record

VA Policy Is Not Optional — It's Legally Binding

Each of the following VA documents enforces these rights internally:

- **38 CFR § 1.579** — Establishes the legal procedures VA must follow for amending records, including forwarding the request to the responsible official, timeframes for reply, and the right to appeal.

- **VA Handbook 6300.4** — Provides the detailed internal process for VA employees. It confirms that all requests for correction **must be reviewed by the originating office** and that the Privacy Officer is responsible for coordinating and tracking the outcome.

- **VHA Directive 1605.01** — Applies these rules specifically to health records maintained by VHA, including CPRS notes, consults, and other documentation. It emphasizes that veterans must be informed in writing of any denial and provided instructions for submitting a disagreement.

Key Point: Nowhere in any of these policies does it say that providers are free to "*decline all changes*" or that the record "*cannot be amended.*" Those are common staff myths — and they're directly contradicted by law.

You Have the Final Word in the Record

Even if the VA denies your amendment request, you are legally entitled to submit a Statement of Disagreement *5 USC § 552a(d)(3)*. This statement:

- Becomes a permanent part of your VA record
- Must be included in every future disclosure of the disputed note
- Cannot be altered or ignored by VA staff

This means you're never powerless. The VA might control what gets written — but you control what gets challenged, clarified, and recorded alongside it.

In the next section, we'll walk through **how to submit a correction request properly** — including where to send it, what to include, and how to avoid common mistakes that lead to delays or denials.

The VA provides a standardized form titled **"Patient Amendment Request"** to help Veterans formally request corrections to their VA health records. This form streamlines the process and ensures that your request is handled according to the rules established in:

- **5 U.S.C. § 552a(d)** (Privacy Act of 1974)
- **38 C.F.R. § 1.579** (Amendment of Records)
- **VA Handbook 6300.4** (Processing of Privacy Act Requests)
- **VHA Directive 1605.01** (Privacy and Release of Information)

This section walks you through each part of the form, what to include, and how to submit it.

Overview: What This Form Does

The Patient Amendment Request Form allows you to:

- Identify exactly what information in your VA record you believe is **inaccurate, incomplete, or misleading**
- Specify **which VA facility** or provider created the record
- Submit **supporting documentation** to justify your request
- Ensure your request is processed by the facility's **Privacy Officer**, as required by law

How to Complete the Form — Section by Section

Top of the Form – Patient Information

Provide your identifying details, including:

- Full name
- Last 4 digits of SSN
- Date of birth
- Address, phone, and email

This information helps ensure your request is matched correctly to your record.

Question 1 – Description of the Record to Be Amended

Be specific about:

- **Which record you want amended** (e.g., "Primary Care note from Dr. Smith states ...")
- **Where it is located** (e.g., "Bay Pines VA Medical Center, under Notes")

Question 2 – Date and Time of the Entry to Be Amended

While the form only asks for the date, **including the time** helps the Privacy Officer locate the record quickly — especially if there are multiple entries on the same day.

Question 3 – Reason for the Amendment Request

Select one or more of the form's suggested reasons:

- The information is inaccurate
- The information is incomplete
- The information is irrelevant
- The information is untimely

Question 4 – How to Correct the Record

State how you want the record to be amended. Be precise. If you already quoted the original statement in Question 1, you do not need to repeat it here. Examples:

- *"Please **delete** the entire statement."*
- *"Please **change** the statement to: '[insert corrected language].'"*
- *"Please **add** after the statement "[missing information"].*

Note: You do not need to explain why the change is necessary here — that explanation should be included in your attached personal statement.

Question 5 – Anyone who may have received or relied on the incorrect information

This is a simple Yes/No question.

- If **No**, you may move on.
- If **Yes**, provide a list of anyone — inside or outside the VA — who may have received or acted on the incorrect information. If you need more space, attach an additional page.

Bottom of the Form

If you are the Veteran, sign and date the form.

If someone is completing the form on your behalf, they must also include:

- Printed Name of Personal Representative
- Representative's Phone Number and mailing address
- Attached proof of legal authority (such as power of attorney, legal guardianship, or official caregiver designation)

Veteran Name: _____ Date: _____

Last 4 SSN: _____   Phone Number: (____) _____

Address: _____
               _____
               _____

1. Description of the information/statement you are requesting to be amended (e.g., health record, lab results): *Attach a copy of record being disputed, if possible.

   _____
   _____
   _____
   _____

2. Date of the information to be amended (*This may be the date of clinic visit, date of the note, procedure or other service): _____

3. What is the reason for requesting this amendment (*Is the information inaccurate, incomplete, irrelevant, or untimely): _____

4. How should the records be stated, *please specify in writing below
   Example 1: Please change statement XYZ to the statement ABC
   Example 2: Please delete the entire statement from my health record

   _____
   _____
   _____
   _____
   _____

5. Do you know of anyone who may have received or relied on the information in question? ☐ Yes   ☐ No   If yes, who? _____

   _____

Signature of Veteran or Personal Representative
* If you are the personal representative, please print your name, address & phone number and attach a copy of relevant legal documenqation (e.g., guardianship, POA, etc.)

Attach a Copy of the Record to be Amended

Include a printed, downloaded, or screenshot copy of the VA medical record entry you want changed. The entry should clearly display:

- The **date and time** of the entry
- The name of the provider who entered it

Appendix G

To avoid confusion, **highlight** the part of the entry you are asking to be amended.

Attach a Personal Statement of Explanation

This is your opportunity to explain **why** the entry is wrong or misleading. Keep it factual and concise. You don't need to cite policy — just clearly explain the error and what the correct record should reflect. Examples:

- *"The note states I refused treatment, but I requested referral to a specialist."*

- *"The problem list does not reflect the diagnosis discussed with me by the provider on [date]."*

- *"The nurse intake note says I exercise three times per week, but I did not say that and I am physically unable to exercise due to my condition."*

Attach Supporting Documentation

Check the appropriate box on the form and include any documents that support your request:

- After Visit Summaries
- Secure Messages
- Past consults or referrals
- Diagnostic test results
- Personal notes or signed witness statements

These attachments increase the strength and credibility of your request.

How to Submit the Form

Send your completed amendment request to the **Privacy Officer** at the VA facility that maintains the record. You can submit it in one of the following ways:

- VA Secure Messenger (recommended)
- **In person** (ask for a date-stamped copy)
- **By mail** (use certified tracking or return receipt)

Every VA Medical Center is required to have a designated Privacy Officer. If you're unsure where to send your form, call the facility's main line or ask the Patient Advocate.

Timelines and What to Expect

VA policy requires the following:

- A written acknowledgment within 10 business days

- A written **decision within 30 business days** (with one allowable 30-day extension)

- If your request is **denied**, the VA must:

    o Provide a written explanation for the denial

    o Explain your right to submit a **Statement of Disagreement**

    o Notify you of your right to appeal to the Office of General Counsel

Keep a Copy of Everything

Make and keep a copy of:

- Your completed amendment request form

- All attachments

- Proof of submission (e.g., mail receipts, screenshots, or stamped copies)

Log all communications and follow-up in your **complaint record**, as described in Appendix E.

Index

VA Structure & Entities

Caregiver Support: 98, 114, 115

clinic: 7, 11, 14, 15, 17, 24, 29, 30, 39, 55, 60, 61, 64, 72, 73, 74, 76, 85, 108, 116, 121, 133, 139, 140, 142, 148, 162, 168, 175, 185

Community Care: 10, 98, 122, 159, 163, 164, 181

facility: 5, 10, 14, 15, 22, 30, 31, 35, 36, 41, 42, 43, 44, 47, 48, 50, 51, 52, 55, 56, 57, 58, 59, 60, 61, 65, 67, 69, 71, 74, 75, 78, 79, 83, 84, 85, 86, 87, 88, 89, 90, 95, 97, 100, 102, 103, 104, 118, 119, 120, 123, 124, 125, 126, 127, 128, 129, 130, 131, 133, 135, 136, 139, 140, 144, 150, 157, 158, 164, 165, 166, 171, 173, 176, 177, 180, 181, 182, 183, 184, 185, 186, 191, 193

medical center: 12, 15, 18, 24, 32, 33, 34, 35, 47, 50, 51, 52, 53, 55, 59, 60, 64, 66, 74, 75, 79, 85, 87, 91, 95, 97, 125, 128, 135, 144, 164, 165, 166, 167, 168, 169, 170, 171, 172, 173, 174, 191, 193

PACT: 9, 11, 67, 69, 117, 119, 124, 128, 134, 135, 136, 137, 138, 139, 140, 141, 142, 143, 144, 145, 157, 161, 163, 165, 166, 184, 185, 186, 187

Patient Advocate: 4, 13, 16, 17, 18, 25, 26, 27, 34, 35, 36, 37, 38, 39, 41, 43, 44, 46, 47, 48, 49, 50, 51, 53, 56, 58, 59, 61, 65, 66, 67, 72, 74, 75, 76, 86, 87, 90, 97, 102, 103, 104, 106, 120, 123, 124, 128, 129, 130, 139, 142, 144, 147, 163, 165, 166, 167, 168, 169, 170, 171, 172, 173, 174, 176, 177, 181, 193

Primary Care: 7, 10, 11, 64, 66, 74, 95, 106, 107, 108, 115, 121, 126, 127, 128, 134, 135, 137, 139, 141, 142, 144, 145, 161, 162, 163, 164, 168, 169, 182, 184, 185, 186, 191

Privacy Officer: 94, 95, 97, 101, 102, 103, 104, 183, 190, 191, 193

VA: 1, 2, 3, 4, 5, 6, 7, 8, 9, 10, 11, 12, 13, 14, 15, 16, 17, 19, 20, 21, 22, 23, 24, 25, 26, 27, 28, 29, 30, 31, 32, 33, 34, 35, 36, 37, 38, 40, 41, 42, 43, 44, 45, 47, 48, 49, 50, 51, 52, 53, 54, 55, 56, 57, 58, 60, 61, 62, 63, 64, 65, 66, 67, 68, 69, 70, 71, 72, 73, 74, 75, 76, 77, 78, 79, 80, 81, 82, 83, 84, 85, 86, 87, 88, 89, 90, 91, 92, 93, 94, 95, 96, 97, 98, 99, 100, 101, 102, 103, 104, 105, 106, 107, 109, 110, 112, 113, 114, 115, 116, 117, 118, 119, 120, 122, 123, 124, 125, 126, 127, 128, 129, 130, 131,

132, 133, 134, 135, 136, 138, 139, 140, 141, 142, 143, 144, 145, 146, 147, 149, 150, 151, 152, 153, 154, 155, 156, 157, 158, 159, 160, 161, 162, 163, 164, 165, 166, 167, 168, 169, 170, 171, 172, 173, 174, 177, 178, 179, 180, 181, 182, 183, 184, 185, 187, 188, 189, 190, 191, 192, 193

VHA: 1, 4, 6, 7, 8, 9, 12, 13, 14, 15, 18, 21, 22, 23, 24, 25, 27, 31, 32, 33, 34, 35, 36, 37, 38, 39, 40, 41, 42, 43, 44, 46, 47, 48, 57, 59, 60, 62, 63, 65, 67, 70, 71, 72, 73, 74, 75, 76, 77, 79, 81, 82, 83, 84, 85, 86, 87, 88, 89, 90, 91, 92, 93, 94, 95, 100, 101, 103, 104, 117, 118, 121, 122, 123, 124, 125, 127, 128, 129, 130, 131, 132, 133, 134, 135, 136, 137, 138, 139, 140, 141, 142, 144, 145, 147, 156, 157, 158, 159, 160, 161, 162, 163, 164, 165, 166, 167, 168, 169, 170, 171, 172, 173, 174, 175, 180, 181, 182, 183, 184, 185, 186, 190

VISN: 15, 24, 26, 32, 35, 44, 47, 48, 50, 51, 52, 53, 55, 56, 58, 59, 60, 65, 67, 71, 72, 73, 74, 75, 76, 77, 79, 90, 102, 103, 104, 131, 139, 144, 150, 157, 164, 165, 167, 168, 169, 171, 172, 173, 174

Legal & Policy References

38 CFR: 13, 29, 30, 31, 32, 92, 93, 94, 189

law: 1, 2, 6, 13, 16, 19, 21, 22, 29, 33, 34, 35, 36, 37, 40, 47, 54, 55, 62, 63, 67, 68, 82, 83, 91, 92, 93, 94, 95, 98, 99, 100, 101, 103, 104, 134, 150, 153, 154, 155, 165, 189, 190, 191

HIPAA: 160, 169, 170, 171, 172

policy: 2, 4, 5, 6, 8, 12, 13, 14, 17, 18, 19, 20, 21, 22, 23, 24, 25, 26, 27, 28, 29, 30, 32, 33, 34, 35, 36, 37, 38, 39, 41, 42, 43, 44, 45, 46, 47, 48, 49, 51, 52, 54, 56, 57, 58, 59, 60, 61, 62, 63, 64, 65, 66, 67, 68, 69, 70, 72, 73, 74, 75, 77, 78, 79, 80, 81, 82, 83, 84, 85, 86, 87, 88, 89, 90, 91, 92, 93, 96, 97, 99, 100, 101, 103, 104, 105, 117, 118, 119, 120, 122, 125, 126, 128, 129, 130, 131, 133, 134, 135, 136, 137, 138, 139, 140, 144, 145, 150, 157, 158, 159, 160, 163, 164, 165, 166, 167, 168, 169, 170, 171, 172, 173, 174, 180, 181, 182, 183, 186, 189, 192, 193

VHA Directive: 13, 14, 18, 21, 22, 23, 24, 27, 31, 32, 34, 35, 36, 37, 38, 39, 40, 41, 42, 43, 44, 46, 47, 48, 57, 59, 60, 62, 65, 67, 70, 71, 72, 73, 75, 76, 77, 79, 81, 82, 83, 84, 85, 86, 87, 88, 89, 90, 91, 92, 93, 94, 95, 100, 101, 103, 104, 117, 118, 121, 122, 123, 124, 125, 127, 128, 129, 130, 131, 132, 133, 147, 156, 157, 158, 159, 160, 161, 162, 163, 164, 165, 166, 167, 168, 169, 170, 171, 172, 173, 174, 175, 180, 181, 183, 190

Complaint & Appeal Mechanisms

appeal: 8, 31, 32, 54, 89, 92, 94, 97, 144, 155, 162, 189, 193

complaint: 3, 4, 12, 13, 15, 17, 18, 23, 24, 25, 26, 27, 30, 31, 32, 33, 34, 35, 36, 37, 40, 41, 44, 47, 48, 49, 50, 51, 52, 54, 55, 56, 57, 58, 59, 60, 61, 62, 63, 64, 65, 66, 67, 68, 69, 70, 71, 72, 73, 74, 75, 76, 77, 78, 79, 80, 86, 88, 89, 90, 91, 97, 101, 102, 103, 123, 124, 129, 131, 134, 138, 139, 140, 141, 142, 144, 145, 146, 147, 150, 153, 154, 155, 158, 165, 166, 167, 168, 169, 170, 171, 172, 173, 174, 176, 181, 193

Congress: 3, 12, 26, 30, 33, 35, 40, 47, 50, 52, 53, 54, 58, 59, 66, 71, 76, 79, 150, 163

escalate: 3, 4, 15, 16, 18, 21, 24, 25, 28, 29, 30, 33, 34, 35, 41, 44, 45, 47, 48, 49, 51, 52, 60, 65, 66, 68, 69, 71, 73, 74, 76, 78, 79, 80, 86, 87, 88, 89, 90, 91, 92, 93, 99, 102, 103, 105, 120, 123, 124, 129, 130, 133, 139, 141, 142, 144, 150, 154, 157, 168, 173, 175

feedback: 13, 14, 41, 155, 180

grievance: 26, 68, 139

OIG: 26, 28, 35, 48, 49, 50, 52, 55, 56, 57, 58, 67, 74, 77, 79, 91, 102, 123, 124, 139, 144, 150, 163, 165, 166, 167, 169, 170, 171, 172, 174

Medical Records

amendment: 79, 81, 92, 93, 94, 95, 97, 98, 100, 102, 103, 104, 105, 106, 107, 112, 115, 147, 154, 155, 162, 170, 171, 175, 178, 179, 187, 188, 189, 190, 191, 193

documentation: 4, 10, 18, 20, 26, 34, 38, 39, 41, 45, 48, 49, 54, 58, 60, 61, 66, 67, 69, 77, 79, 80, 81, 82, 85, 91, 92, 94, 95, 97, 98, 100, 104, 106, 108, 109, 110, 115, 144, 145, 147, 148, 154, 159, 161, 162, 163, 164, 166, 167, 169, 170, 172, 173, 174, 181, 190, 191, 192

entry: 34, 93, 95, 96, 98, 99, 101, 104, 109, 110, 111, 115, 153, 170, 171, 172, 181, 189, 191, 192

error: 96, 98, 103, 113, 192

medical record: 79, 81, 83, 92, 93, 96, 101, 102, 105, 111, 112, 115, 116, 147, 154, 169, 170, 171, 172, 183, 192

notation: 154

Access & Treatment Issues

access: 4, 9, 10, 16, 22, 23, 30, 32, 39, 41, 42, 55, 64, 65, 66, 67, 74, 81, 82, 84, 86, 91, 98, 117, 118, 119, 120, 121, 123, 125, 127, 129, 130, 131, 134, 135, 136, 137, 138, 139, 140, 143, 144, 145, 147, 154, 158, 159, 160, 161, 162, 163, 166, 168, 173, 178, 180, 183, 185, 186, 187, 189

appointment: 5, 10, 26, 30, 46, 62, 64, 66, 107, 108, 111, 119, 136, 137, 139, 144, 164, 167, 168, 169, 186

care coordination: 119, 120, 147, 161, 168, 169, 185, 187

continuity of care: 60, 121, 135, 136, 137, 139, 140, 141, 144, 185, 186

chronic: 11, 122, 124, 135, 138, 141, 183

delay: 36, 46, 47, 49, 57, 61, 62, 65, 66, 67, 70, 72, 74, 78, 83, 85, 90, 91, 105, 114, 115, 116, 121, 128, 130, 132, 155, 159, 161, 166, 167, 168, 169

denial: 55, 62, 65, 88, 90, 94, 97, 99, 100, 101, 102, 103, 104, 106, 115, 128, 129, 130, 155, 162, 172, 173, 174, 188, 190, 193

follow-up: 27, 35, 38, 41, 51, 52, 59, 61, 62, 64, 65, 69, 70, 71, 72, 73, 77, 89, 97, 103, 108, 110, 121, 122, 124, 126, 130, 134, 137, 138, 142, 143, 157, 161, 170, 180, 193

referral: 10, 11, 15, 17, 27, 31, 38, 46, 62, 63, 64, 72, 74, 89, 96, 99, 119, 120, 121, 124, 128, 167, 168, 169, 181, 192

scheduling: 30, 64, 65, 77, 131, 135, 142, 157, 167, 168, 169

treatment: 16, 59, 65, 96, 98, 107, 108, 109, 111, 112, 113, 116, 120, 122, 125, 126, 127, 138, 158, 160, 185, 192

waitlist: 130, 141

Veteran Experience

chronic: 11, 122, 124, 135, 138, 141, 183

disability: 2, 5, 8, 9, 21, 24, 26, 54, 55, 81, 82, 83, 84, 87, 89, 98, 114, 156, 159, 163, 164, 172, 173, 174, 179, 182

eligibility: 9, 98, 105, 109, 114, 115, 121, 156, 162

mental health: 87, 98, 99, 118, 121, 127, 156, 162, 164, 182

mobility: 109, 113

pain: 109, 110, 111, 113, 114, 148, 152

physical: 54, 107, 114, 115

rating: 2, 5, 10, 54, 110

service-connected: 9, 64, 98

trauma: 98, 99, 158

VA benefits: 54, 159, 182

Forms & Communication

communication: 9, 11, 14, 17, 22, 26, 27, 28, 38, 40, 41, 42, 43, 45, 54, 57, 60, 62, 63, 65, 70, 77, 88, 89, 113, 118, 121, 138, 140, 142, 143, 144, 145, 147, 155, 161, 167, 168, 187

email: 18, 44, 48, 52, 54, 67, 69, 74, 76, 95, 130, 165, 166, 175, 191

form: 1, 3, 21, 23, 44, 48, 54, 70, 74, 81, 82, 83, 84, 85, 86, 87, 88, 89, 90, 92, 93, 95, 96, 97, 98, 101, 109, 113, 127, 138, 148, 149, 156, 159, 161, 163, 172, 173, 182, 183, 190, 191, 192, 193

MyHealtheVet: 26, 44, 46, 72, 76, 88, 119, 129, 139, 140, 142, 163, 164, 175

phone: 10, 24, 26, 30, 57, 64, 67, 69, 73, 89, 95, 96, 114, 119, 131, 137, 138, 144, 165, 166, 191, 192

Accountability & Oversight

accountability: 5, 15, 21, 24, 26, 27, 28, 33, 34, 35, 36, 46, 47, 52, 53, 54, 58, 59, 60, 61, 63, 69, 71, 73, 75, 79, 82, 102, 123, 124, 133, 144, 145, 149, 151, 152, 153, 155, 156, 157, 161, 171

case manager: 163

Director: 12, 15, 18, 24, 26, 40, 42, 44, 48, 50, 51, 58, 59, 60, 65, 67, 71, 74, 75, 77, 79, 123, 124, 131, 139, 144, 165, 167, 168, 169, 170, 171, 172, 173, 174, 176, 182, 183

leadership: 14, 15, 16, 21, 25, 27, 31, 34, 35, 36, 38, 41, 44, 45, 47, 48, 49, 51, 52, 53, 54, 56, 59, 60, 61, 65, 66, 67, 69, 72, 73, 74, 75, 76, 77, 79, 80, 82, 86, 90, 102, 103, 122, 125, 133, 144, 149, 150, 151, 155, 157, 158, 163, 164, 165, 166, 167, 168, 169, 171, 172, 173, 175, 177

Supervisor: 34, 35, 41, 43, 44, 47, 53, 56, 59, 72, 73, 74, 75, 119, 139, 165, 167, 168, 169, 170, 171, 172, 181

About the Author

John Lafferty is a disabled veteran, former enlisted Marine, and former U.S. Navy Civil Engineer Corps Officer who brings contract law expertise, engineering discipline, and lived experience to the fight for VA accountability. Trained in federal contracting, he led multimillion-dollar construction and facility support projects during his Navy service — experience that now shapes his advocacy for Veterans navigating the complex VA health care system.

After his military service, John became a data science lead at Booz Allen Hamilton, where he helped transform government operations through analytics and automation. Following his departure from the workforce due to service-connected conditions, he began a new mission: confronting the systemic failures Veterans face — from inaccurate records to ignored complaints and policy violations.

Navigating VA Health Care is the result — a practical, plain-language guide that empowers Veterans to push back with evidence, not emotion, and to demand the care they've earned.

Made in the USA
Columbia, SC
05 August 2025

b478ab37-9b11-4e72-8e76-b385307e8b65R01